Become the mom
you want to be

[signature]

BECOMING **MUM**

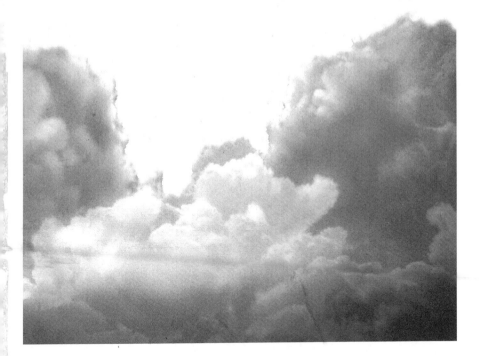

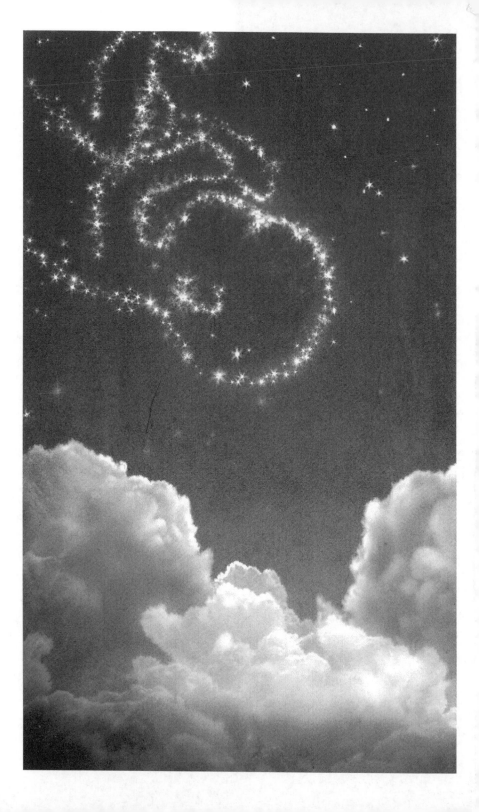

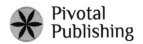
Pivotal
Publishing

DR **KOA WHITTINGHAM**
BECOMING **MUM**

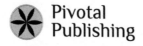

Pivotal
Publishing

Pivotal Publishing Pty Ltd
pivotalpublishing.com.au
Brisbane, Australia

Becoming Mum
AUTHOR
DESIGNER

Copyright © 2013, Dr Koa Whittingham
Dr Koa Whittingham, *koawhittingham.com*
Stuart Gibson, *bookdesign.com.au*
Cover imagery courtesy of *istock.com*

First published 2013   10 9 8 7 6 5 4 3 2 1

National Library of Australia Cataloguing-in-Publication entry

AUTHOR
TITLE
ISBN
SUBJECTS

DEWEY NUMBER

Whittingham,Koa, author.
Becoming Mum/ Dr Koa Whittingham.
978-0-9922726-0-9 (paperback).
Motherhood—Psychological aspects.
Mothers—Psychology.
Pregnancy—Psychological aspects.
Mother and child—Psychological aspects.
306.8743

Contents

What is *Becoming Mum* all about?   **i**

1   **What do I value as a mother?**   **1**

Values: your guiding stars 2
Exploring your mothering values 3
One woman's story 7
My unique adventure 9
Putting it into practice 12

2   **Motherhood and pain**   **14**

Suffering and joy are attached 15
Fighting an unwinnable battle 16
The struggle and becoming a mum 20
Letting go of the struggle 22
One woman's story 23
My unique adventure 24
Putting it into practice 26

3   **Living with monsters**   **27**

Meet the monsters 28
Seeing the monsters in broad daylight 32
Where do my monsters come from? 33
Living with monsters 33
Monster radio 34
One woman's story 37
My unique adventure 38
Putting it into practice 40

4   Mindfulness   41

What is mindfulness? 41
A taste of mindfulness 42
Mindfulness of breathing 44
Mindful walking 48
Developing a regular mindfulness practice 50
Waking up *(Mindfulness in everyday life)* 52
One woman's story 52
My unique adventure 54
Putting it into practice 55

5   Mindful mothering   56

What is mindful mothering? 56
Mindfulness of baby during pregnancy 57
Mindfulness of baby 59
Waking up to baby *(Mindfulness of baby in everyday life)* . . 62
One woman's story 63
My unique adventure 65
Putting it into practice 67

6   Thoughts are just thoughts   68

Getting caught in our thoughts 68
Mindfulness of thoughts 71
Noticing thoughts as thoughts in everyday life 73
One woman's story 76
My unique adventure 77
Putting it into practice 79

7   The emotional journey   80

Mindfulness of emotions 81
Emotions in daily life 85
My emotions, baby's emotions 87
One woman's story 89
My unique adventure 91
Putting it into practice 94

8 **When the here & now is physically painful** **95**

Mindfulness and physical pain or discomfort 95
Living through it 98
Draw strength from your values. 99
Be kind to yourself 101
One woman's story 101
My unique adventure 103
Putting it into practice 104

9 **Loving baby** **105**

What is a mother's love? 105
Becoming an accepting space for your baby 107
Kindness for baby 111
Love in action 113
A developing bond. 114
One woman's story 115
My unique adventure 117
Putting it into practice 120

10 **Taking care of yourself** **121**

Taking care of yourself is taking care of your baby . 122
Kindness for self, kindness for baby 123
Self-kindness in daily life 126
Acts of self-kindness 127
Accepting our mistakes 128
Settling baby, settling self. 129
One woman's story 131
My unique adventure 133
Putting it into practice 135

11 **Building a rewarding life** **136**

Why a rewarding life is important 136
Values as guiding stars 137
Building a rewarding life while trying to conceive . 139
Building a rewarding life for pregnancy 140

Building a rewarding life for a new mum 141
Scheduling your life 143
Think small—really small 146
Building your rewarding life 147
One woman's story 149
My unique adventure 151
Putting it into practice 152

12 **Social support**   **154**
My values in relation to family and friendships . . 154
Surveying my social world 157
Building positive relationships 161
Effective communication. 162
Ignore the bad and reward the good 164
Improving social support. 165
One woman's story 174
My unique adventure 176
Putting it into practice 178

13 **Changes in your romantic relationship**   **180**
Two journeys, taken together 180
The relationship matters to baby 183
Values in the relationship 183
Building a positive relationship 185
Ignore the bad, reward the good 185
Continuing to nourish your relationship 186
Sex and nourishing your relationship 188
Parenting together 189
What if my partner just isn't playing the game? . . 191
One woman's story 193
My unique adventure 195
Putting it into practice 197

14 **Returning to values** **199**

Your unique mothering values 199
Greater clarity 202
Understanding your newborn baby 203
The implications of my values 207
Goals for now 212
One woman's story 213
My unique adventure 216
Putting it into practice 217

15 **Acting on mothering values** **218**

And here come the monsters 218
Small acts for here and now 222
Expect to slip 223
Do what works in becoming the
    mum you want to be 224
Actually doing it 225
One woman's story 226
My unique adventure 227
Putting it into practice 229

16 **In a nutshell** **230**

This is your adventure 230
The journey in a moment 231
Take this lightly too! 233
And finally 233
A poem for baby 234
A second poem for baby 234

What is the research behind this book? **235**

References **239**

About the author **242**

To my darling daughter and to my little ones yet to be.

What is
Becoming Mum
all about?

Becoming a mother is undoubtedly one of the biggest and most important transitions of a woman's life. It is a transition filled with joy, sorrow, doubt and anxiety. It is also a transition that includes dramatic physical challenges, from morning sickness to the birth itself. Further, it is a transition that has wide-reaching flow-on effects, changing a woman's relationship with her partner, her career, her family and her friends. It may even change a woman's fundamental ideas about her own life.

These changes may be welcomed, liberating and joyful, or they may be scary or associated with loss. For many women, the changes are both joyful and nerve-wracking at the very same time. Of course, this is if everything goes smoothly and according to plan. The journey to motherhood can also include additional challenges such as unplanned pregnancy, infertility, complications in pregnancy, miscarriage, preterm birth or postnatal depression. It can also bring into sharp relief pre-existing difficulties such as relationship problems, unresolved family difficulties or personal challenges such as perfectionism, anxiety or low self-esteem. Women may feel under sudden pressure to have these difficulties fixed, quickly, now, before baby arrives.

You may be wondering just how you are going to cope with all of these challenges. How are you going to get through it all and remain, or even become, happy and well adjusted? How are you going to cope with the changes and still maintain what's important to you in your life? Then, on top of all of that, how are you going to be a good mum—and just what is a good mum anyway? What kind of mum do *you* want to be?

If you are finding yourself asking these questions, then this is the book for you.

There already exist numerous excellent books with clear information on the physical realities of conception, pregnancy and birth. In addition, there are many excellent books with practical advice on caring for your newborn child. This book is for the other aspects of the journey, the *psychological* passage to motherhood. I'd encourage you to still access books on conception, pregnancy, birth and caring for your baby, but I hope that this book will support your psychological transformation. I hope that within this book you'll find practical solutions to the problems of how to cope with the challenges that you are facing, how to turn this transition into an experience of psychological growth and how to come out the other end being the kind of mum that you want to be.

This book is based on the latest developments in Cognitive Behavioural Therapy (CBT), including mindfulness-based CBT and Acceptance and Commitment Therapy (ACT, said as one word: 'act'). CBT has an extensive evidence base, and evidence for the newest developments in CBT, including mindfulness-based CBT and ACT, is growing fast. (For more information on the research behind this book, please see the section at the end of the book.) I'd like to acknowledge the many researchers and clinicians whose work in the area of CBT and ACT, as well as in child development and parenting, has provided the firm foundation on which this book was written. *Becoming Mum* began as a glimmer of an idea while I was trying to conceive my first pregnancy. As a clinical and developmental psychologist, I wondered why a book based on the best current research in order to give women—all women—psychological support on the journey to motherhood did not exist. *Becoming Mum* grew into a clear idea by the end of my pregnancy, and writing an outline became a way of occupying myself while heavily pregnant, over my due date and not so patiently awaiting the beginning of labour. Much of this book was, quite literally, written on a laptop propped up on my knees while my newborn baby slept curled in a little ball on my chest. I think this makes *Becoming Mum* a sincere and genuine book. I hope that you think so too.

Becoming Mum is organised into chapters based on psychological content (that is, topics and skills) rather than stages of the process. The book as a whole is intended to be relevant to women at any stage, whether you are currently trying to conceive, pregnant, or the mother of a young baby. As you progress on your journey, you may find that you return to specific chapters or exercises as they become more relevant to you.

In addition, *Becoming Mum* is written to be flexible to your unique circumstances and experiences. This is achieved by organising each chapter into four sections. In the first section the ideas presented in the chapter will be explored, as well as being illustrated by specific exercises and strategies along the way. Space is provided after the exercises so that you can note your own responses to the exercise. I'd encourage you to read this book with a pen in hand, jotting down your responses as you go in order to get the most out of this book. I have alternated between referring to your baby as 'she' and 'he' throughout in order to avoid gender biased language in a way that is still easy to read and has a personal feel.

The second section is called '*One woman's story*', and in this section the content of the chapter is related to the life of one woman. If you are unsure about the concepts or exercises in a chapter, then reading '*One woman's story*' may help you to gain clarity. In addition, you may find that you relate to some of the experiences discussed, and this may make it easier to apply the ideas to your own life.

In the third section, '*My unique adventure*', specific comments will be made to help you relate the content in the chapter to your own personal experiences. Suggestions on how to relate the material to specific circumstances will be made throughout the book as relevant. Thus, you might find your circumstances highlighted and commented on in some chapters but not in others.

The final section in every chapter is '*Putting it into practice*', where practical suggestions will be made on how to apply the content of the chapter to your own life. I hope you find *Becoming Mum* a useful companion. All the best on your journey.

1

What do I value as a mother?

Becoming a mother is undoubtedly one of the most important events in a woman's life. Many women state that becoming a mum is their most significant achievement, their greatest source of satisfaction and fulfilment and their greatest source of joy. You may even feel this already.

If you are reading this book then you are embarking on the wondrous adventure of becoming a mum. It may be that you are currently trying to conceive, or are pregnant, or are the mother of a newborn baby. You may have set out on this journey intentionally—perhaps becoming a mum is something you always knew you wanted to do—or perhaps the adventure has begun unexpectedly. Alternatively, you may be embarking on the journey to motherhood for a second (or third, or fourth . . .) time. Regardless of your situation, you are now making one of the most important transitions of your life. Although this transition will bring many challenges, it is important that we begin not by focusing on how you'll cope with these challenges, but instead by understanding the kind of mum you want to be.

The best way to begin a journey is by knowing your desired destination; otherwise you are likely to end up somewhere else entirely. So let's begin by exploring your destination: you becoming the mum that you want to be. This will mean understanding the values that you have as a mother and the ways in which being a mum can bring satisfaction and fulfilment to your life. In this chapter we'll introduce the concept of values and begin to explore your unique values as a mum. Becoming a mother isn't just challenging; it also has the potential to be deeply fulfilling. By exploring what becoming a mum means to you, you'll have a clearer sense of how to make the transition to motherhood a fulfilling experience. Furthermore, a better sense of what becoming a mum means to you will give you strength to face the challenges that arise and the confidence to make day-to-day decisions as a mother.

VALUES: YOUR GUIDING STARS

Our personal values are the things that we deeply care about, the things that give our lives meaning and purpose and the things that we genuinely enjoy. Our values are what we really want, deep down, our lives to be about. Our own values are personal and unique to us. It is important to understand that our values can't be right or wrong; they simply matter to us. When we put our values at the centre of our lives and use them to guide our day-to-day decisions, our lives become meaningful, fulfilling and enriching.

Your parenting values will be your guiding stars throughout your parenting adventure. Long before GPS, sailors relied upon celestial navigation to cross the oceans and sail to distant lands. They would use celestial objects such as the sun, moon and stars to calculate their position and to guide the journey. In the same way, you'll use your unique mothering values as a mum to guide your own journey. These values include the key aspects of mothering that matter to you, the qualities you want to demonstrate as a mum and the ways in which mothering brings you joy and fulfilment.

Before we begin to explore your values, it is important to understand some additional concepts about values:

✿ Our values underpin the goals that we make, but they aren't goals; they are bigger than that. A goal can be achieved. For example, a mum might have the goal of singing her baby a lullaby tonight, and once she has sung the lullaby, that goal is achieved. However, the mother's goal may be underpinned by a *value* of encouraging musical development. This aim is a value because it can never be fully reached: there's always more encouraging to do!

✿ Values, unlike goals, are flexible to changes in our circumstances. If we have a clear sense of the values that underpin our plans and goals, then, when our plans are thwarted and need to be changed, it is easier to be flexible and to know how we can still live out our values as best we can.

✿ Values come from the heart. Following our values means doing what is important to us, irrespective of whether other people approve or not. Although doing so will not always be easy, it will often give us a sense of satisfaction or a 'just right' feeling of having done what matters to us.

✿ Our values, just like a guiding star, can guide us through stormy seas. There is a dignity and strength in choosing to face something painful, difficult or frightening in the service of something important to us.

In spite of how important values are, we often don't spend much time explicitly thinking about them. You may even find that, right now, you aren't entirely certain what your values as a mum are. So let's begin to explore your mothering values with some thought experiments.

EXPLORING YOUR MOTHERING VALUES

Imagine being able, unseen and unheard, to watch and hear your child (or your future child if you are trying to conceive) as an adult, 20 or 30 years in the future. In your mind's eye, allow yourself to imagine your child, all grown up, going about his or her daily life. What do you wish for him? What do you hope him to be like? What characteristics do you hope to have fostered in him? See your child interacting with workmates and friends; imagine him in love; imagine him interacting with his own children. Write down your thoughts here.

I want to encourage my child to grow into an adult who is:

....

....

....

....

....

....

....

Imagine that your child shows those exact characteristics that you are hoping to encourage. Consider what actions you may have taken as a mother to have encouraged these characteristics in your child.

As a mother, I may have contributed to the development of my child's characteristics by:

....

....

....

....

....

....

....

Now imagine that you are watching your child, as an adult, reflect on his own childhood. Perhaps you might like to imagine that he is talking about his childhood with a partner or with a friend. What memories of his childhood do you hope to hear him recall? Imagine that he begins discussing you, as a mother.

What would you hope to hear him say about you? You probably would love to hear him say that you were a good mother, but try to push past that to the specifics. Imagine him completing one of the following sentences: 'The thing that's really special about my mum is . . . ' or 'I'll always be grateful to my mum for . . . ' or 'I'm lucky I had the mum I had because . . . '.

The impression I want to leave on my child is one of . . .

....

....

....

....

....

....

....

Now imagine that you are transported from Earth to a special, magical place with your child. In this special place it is just you and your child as a newborn baby. If you are currently trying to conceive or are pregnant, imagine that in this magical place you are with your child as a newborn or as a young baby. There is no one else here to judge you and no pressure to achieve anything in particular as a mother. Your baby is alert and calm. Your baby is just happy to be with you and doesn't need anything in particular right now. Somehow you just know that in this special, magical place you can do whatever you want as a mother, with the guarantee that no harm will come to your baby. You are both completely protected, so there is no pressure to get anything right. This is just a special time for you to *enjoy* your baby. If you could simply *enjoy* being a mum without the need to do anything 'right', without fear of judgment from others, without pressure from the outside world or from baby's needs, what would you do?

As a mother, I enjoy (or imagine I will enjoy) my baby by:

....

....

....

....

....

....

....

Now look over your answers to the thought experiments above, and compare them to the earlier description of what values are. Remember that your values come from your heart, are the core things that matter to you and are bigger than goals. Unlike goals, which can be achieved, there's always more to do in living out your values. For example, no matter how many hugs you give your baby, if you have a value of being a loving, affectionate mum there are always more hugs to give.

As you look through your answers you may find that some of the responses you have given are goals rather than values. If so, see if you can identify the value underlying the goal.

How would you summarise your values as a mum? Take a moment to write down your key values here:

....

....

....

....

....

....

....

Now that you have a sense of what your values are as a mum, you can put your values at the centre of your life. As we move on in the next chapter to explore the challenges involved in becoming a mother, it is important to remember that the reason you are facing these challenges is so that you can become the mum you want to be. Further, your values provide the bedrock for the daily decisions that you will have to make as a mum. Thus, having a clearer sense of your own values will bring greater confidence in making these decisions. Putting your values at the centre of your life doesn't mean that life will always be easy or that you'll always feel happy. But it does mean that your life, even when it is difficult, will be fulfilling, enriching and the life you want to live.

If you still feel unsure about what your values as a mum are, that is okay. They will become clearer to you over time. It is common to discover your parenting values after you take your baby home. Pay particular attention to actions that bring you a sense of joy and fulfilment as a mum, as it is likely that these actions are driven by your values. Don't worry, though, if you are still feeling unsure about how to live your life based on your values in a concrete, day-to-day sense—we will be exploring this in detail in future chapters.

ONE WOMAN'S STORY
Reading Akira's story may help you in discovering your own parenting values.
When Akira unexpectedly fell pregnant several years earlier than she and her partner, Jonathon had planned, they were both delighted. Although the pregnancy was a surprise, for Akira it was a happy surprise. However, she quickly became anxious about becoming a mum and fearful that she wouldn't be good at it. In fact, Akira would be the first to admit that she lacked confidence in general. In spite of frequent reassurances from Jonathon and her friends, she often felt that she wasn't good enough for them. She realised that this was probably due to her experiences in her own family. Akira was an only child

and her mum was frequently critical of her. As a child, Akira had felt that she never really lived up to her mother's expectations. Akira was determined to not repeat these mistakes with her own children. She wanted to be a different kind of mum.

Throughout her pregnancy, Akira read many books on pregnancy and caring for babies, spent time on parenting forums on the internet and picked the brains of friends and family. In spite of all of this searching, Akira still felt confused and riddled with self-doubt. It didn't help that much of the advice was contradictory. Akira's cousin gave her long talks on the importance of a completely natural birth while her friends assured her that if she didn't take the drugs she'd be in agony. Her grandmother explained how important it was to create a routine with feeding and sleeping and to be strict with putting the baby to bed in her own cot from the very beginning. Yet, her cousin insisted that the baby must sleep in the same bed as Akira or else she would grow up to be an 'emotional cripple', while her friends shrugged at this debate and said, 'whatever gets you sleep'. The advice from Akira's mother was, as always, highly critical of whatever Akira did or planned to do. Once baby Tilly was born, Akira found herself mulling over all of her actions, anxiously wondering whether she was doing the wrong thing.

After spending some time considering her own values as a mum, Akira felt that what really mattered the most to her was that baby Tilly knew that she was loved unconditionally. Akira wanted to be a loving, caring mum. She also realised that she wanted her baby to grow into an adult who had good self-esteem and confidence. She felt that, as a mum, she could encourage her baby to feel loved and valued by responding to her baby's needs, listening to what her baby had to say (crying, babbling and nonverbal signals) and giving her baby plenty of physical affection. When Akira reflected on how she enjoyed baby Tilly, she realised that she loved being physically affectionate with her. In fact, she liked nothing more than spending time simply cuddling her baby. Akira realised that she could allow herself to enjoy physical closeness with her baby. She also realised that, as she herself loved singing and painting, she wanted to encourage her baby to be a creative, well-rounded person. Akira decided to encourage this by singing her baby lots of lullabies and songs.

Akira discussed her mothering values with Jonathon and they talked about how they wanted to parent together. This allowed Akira to sift through all of the advice that she had been given and pick out that which suited her best. It also helped her to cope with her mother's criticism because Akira now recognised that she was mothering in the way that mattered to her.

MY UNIQUE ADVENTURE

These comments may help you to understand how the information in this chapter might relate to your own unique experiences.

Becoming a confident mum

May be relevant to women at any stage who are struggling to find confidence in their own mothering, coping with self-doubt or coping with criticism and advice from others.

Many women find it difficult to develop confidence as a mum. Often women begin the voyage to motherhood with little experience in or knowledge of pregnancy and caring for a newborn baby. Relatives and friends may be flooding you with advice. This advice may be useful and helpful, but it can also be critical, out of date, forcefully delivered ('you must . . . '), inappropriate for your own life, inappropriate for your baby, or inconsistent with your unique values as a mum. This may be the case even with kindly meant advice given with every good intention. This can contribute to your self-doubts and confusion.

The values that you hold as a mum are the foundation on which you can make plans, set goals or decide the way that is best, for both you and your baby, to meet any challenges that you experience. Therefore, the clearer your values are to you, the easier it is to separate the advice that's useful from the advice that is not best for you. When considering the advice of others, ask yourself if it fits with your mothering style. Remember that while the advice may be kindly meant, it may be based on values that are different from yours. So, when making a mothering decision, look at the options in light of your values. Which action is consistent with being the mum you want to be?

Becoming Mum ... again
May be relevant to women with older children who are pregnant or have a new baby

If you have older children, your experiences with mothering them may have given you a clearer sense of your mothering values. Perhaps you are confident about what you want to do this time around. Alternatively, you may have slipped into crisis mode and lost touch with what is important to you as a parent. Regardless, repeat the exercises in this chapter while thinking about your older children as well as your new baby. What kind of mother do you want to be to them? Notice the times when you enjoy being a mother to your older children. What are you doing? What does this tell you about your parenting values? What small action can you take, today, to be the kind of mother you want to be to your older children too?

Reversing the downward spiral
May be relevant to women with a history of depression, at risk of postnatal depression or experiencing postnatal depression.

In preventing and combating depression it is particularly important to ask yourself how you enjoy your baby. Reconnect with the values around motherhood that give you that 'just right' feeling. If you are currently experiencing depression, you may not be enjoying anything right now. Still, start doing the mothering actions that you would normally enjoy even if they don't currently bring enjoyment. With time, the enjoyment often begins to appear.

Help! This wasn't what I had planned!

May be relevant to women experiencing difficulty conceiving, miscarriage, complications, preterm birth, an unwanted birth experience or finding motherhood different from expectations.
Unfortunately life, including motherhood, doesn't always happen according to plan. It is not unusual for our most prized, best-laid plans to be unexpectedly thwarted. It is, of course, completely natural and healthy to experience disappointment, sadness, anger or grief in these circumstances. However, if you have a clear sense of the values that underpin your plan it is easier to adapt to the new circumstances and to find ways of continuing to live your values. Of course, this doesn't mean that you won't still grieve or be disappointed. But it does mean that it'll be easier to find what you can do in the circumstances to be the mum you want to be.

Read through your mothering values and ask yourself, is there an action that I can take today, however small, to fulfil these values? In your circumstances you may need to be creative in how you fulfil this value. For example, you may value being a loving, affectionate mother. What can you do towards this value when you are trying to conceive, or after a miscarriage, or if your baby is in neonatal intensive care? Consider all the ways that you could express love for your baby: through words or song, by making her something, by writing her a letter. Find a small action that you can take today and take it. Notice the effect that this has on you.

How do I survive this?

May be relevant to women experiencing emotional challenges, tough physical symptoms such as morning sickness, or birth.
There's a big difference between being the unwilling victim of circumstance and facing an emotional or physical challenge because it is a part of being the mum that you want to be. Many a woman has taken a deep breath, said to herself, 'I'm doing this for my baby', and found that it has made all

the difference. Use your values as guides to lead you through the challenges. You might like to write your values down and put them somewhere visible to remind yourself every day why you are facing the challenges that you are facing. You might also like to develop mantras for the difficult times, based on your values. Even something as simple as 'I'm doing this for my baby' has great power.

Young mums and unplanned pregnancies

May be relevant to young mothers, younger-than-planned mothers and women experiencing an unplanned pregnancy.

If you are a young mum or if you are experiencing an unplanned pregnancy (a pregnancy that perhaps happened earlier than you had planned or a pregnancy that wasn't in your life plans at all) then it is doubly important for you to spend time reflecting now on your values as a mother. You may find it helpful to talk to other women about their values as mums, particularly women in a similar situation to you or women who were in a similar situation to you and are now confident mums of toddlers or young children. You may find that it takes time for you to get a good sense of your own values as a mum. This is fine. Remember, women who are experiencing a pregnancy that has been planned and/or that is occurring later in life have had plenty of time to reflect on becoming a mother before they fell pregnant. What is important is to give yourself the time and space to reflect on becoming a mum now.

PUTTING IT INTO PRACTICE

- ✰ Write your values down and put them somewhere that you see every day to remind yourself why you are facing the challenges that you are facing.
- ✰ Do something small, today, to live out your values as a mum. If you are still trying to conceive, you may need to be creative; for example, consider ways that you can express your love for your baby now, such as writing your baby a letter or making something for your baby. Perhaps there are actions

you can take now to prepare for your future baby, such as learning to sing a particular lullaby? If you have experienced a miscarriage, consider whether there is something that you can do as a mum for your lost baby. This may be as simple as planting a tree in your garden or lighting a candle. It should be a gesture that holds meaning for you.

☆ Talk to other women about their values as mums. Are their values similar to or different from yours? Considering how your values are similar to or different from theirs may also help you to evaluate how relevant their advice may be to your situation.

☆ Notice times when, as a mum, you feel a joyous, 'just right' feeling. It is likely that at these times you are acting on your values. What are you doing? What value are you acting on?

2

Motherhood
and pain

Motherhood is the perfect life experience for discovering a key insight into human life. That insight is this: suffering and joy are attached. They are, in fact, two sides of the same coin. It is no coincidence, then, that becoming a mum is filled with both joy *and* suffering. No wonder many women find the transition to motherhood stressful and challenging! Unfortunately, we often forget this fact and try to eliminate our emotional pain. In doing so we are really fighting a battle with ourselves, with our own thoughts, feelings and memories. This is both an unwinnable battle and a distraction from vital, meaningful living.

In this chapter we will explore why joy and emotional pain are attached, and how we relate to the suffering we experience. You will be encouraged to think of your emotional pain in a different way. Instead of seeing it as something to be fought and eliminated, you'll be encouraged to let go of the struggle with your own pain and instead expend your energy on becoming the mum you want to be. This may be a very different way of thinking of suffering for you, so I'd encourage you to digest the information in this chapter slowly, allowing yourself to really understand why letting go of the struggle may be the

best thing to do. In future chapters, we'll explore exactly how
to let go of the struggle in a concrete way.

SUFFERING AND JOY ARE ATTACHED

It seems that it is a universal feature of the human condition
that emotional suffering and joy are two sides of the same
coin. It is impossible to love without opening yourself up to
heartbreak, impossible to succeed without facing failure or
fear of failure, impossible to build a joyful existence without
creating the possibility of losing it. Likewise, attempts to rid
our lives of emotional pain (and this includes sadness, fear
or anxiety) also strip our lives of joy, happiness and love. Our
pain and our joy go hand in hand. It seems that we can either
live our lives abundantly, with hearts and minds flung wide
open to life, or we can measure our lives out carefully, tiptoe-
ing around our emotional pain but missing out on joy as well.
But don't take my word for it. See for yourself whether this is
true of your own life.

Take a moment to consider the emotional suffering in your
life. This may include sadness, fear, anxiety or anger. Consider
not only any emotional pain associated with motherhood but
also emotional suffering in other areas of your life as well. List
your biggest sources of emotional pain here.

What are some of your saddest moments? Your biggest fears?
Your greatest anxieties? Your biggest sources of anger?

....

....

....

....

....

....

....

And are those sad moments, those big fears, those moments of anger, attached to something else? Are they, in fact, attached to the very things that matter most to you in life? Are they attached to your greatest sources of joy, your most precious dreams and your values? After all, why would you worry so much about being a good mum if being a good mum wasn't deeply important to you? Would you fear losing your baby if you didn't love your baby deeply? Would you feel sadness when you make a mistake as a mum if you didn't passionately care about being the mum you want to be?

Take a moment to think through how your suffering relates to your values and your joy and write down your thoughts here.

....

....

....

....

....

....

....

You aren't alone. But what are the implications of this insight?

FIGHTING AN UNWINNABLE BATTLE

Unfortunately, our minds don't always see that our pain and our joy are two sides of the very same coin. Instead, we often find ourselves trying to have the joy without the suffering. You may have noticed yourself trying to experience just the joy associated with becoming a mum without the worry, sadness, anger or fear that is also associated with this transition. Perhaps you've even thought that you *should* experience only joy when becoming a mother; that somehow the worries, fears, anger or sadness are wrong and must be eliminated for you to become a mum in the right way. 'What's wrong with wanting to experience only joy?' you may ask. Surely it would be better to cut away the pain and just leave the joy?

Of course, absolutely nothing is wrong with taking steps to eliminate or lessen our suffering, so long as it works and we don't accidentally cut away the joy in the process. Unfortunately, however, because our joy and our pain are attached at a deep level, it just isn't possible to truly eliminate our suffering completely. Although we can sometimes take steps to lessen it without sacrificing what we hold dear, we are never truly free of it.

There are good reasons why our attempts to eliminate our emotional pain ultimately fall short of their goal. Our attempts are really struggles with our own emotions, thoughts and memories. In other words, when we get caught in a struggle to eliminate our emotional suffering we are really caught in a struggle with ourselves. It shouldn't be a surprise that struggling with ourselves—with the issues in our own minds and hearts—doesn't work. However, we tend to think it will because the strategies that we use often work so well with the external problems we deal with out there in the world.

Imagine that after putting this book down you take a walk around your house and notice a particular picture hanging on the wall. You decide that you don't like this picture anymore. Could you get rid of it? Of course you could. In fact, taking the picture down from the wall and destroying it is relatively easy. Now imagine that as you take a walk around your house you notice a particular memory. You decide that you don't like this memory any more. Could you get rid of it? This is not so easy: you can't just get rid of the memory in the same way that you could get rid of the picture. You could possibly distract yourself for a while, but the memory is still there. All it would take is for someone to say, 'Hey, remember when . . . ', and bam, it would be back again. Unfortunately, we are often so successful at getting rid of what we don't want in the external world that it is very tempting to think we could simply get rid of unwanted 'internal stuff' too.

Let's try another thought experiment. This one is really very simple. In a moment you'll read 'Ready, Steady, Go!'. When you read this, pause and sit still for one minute. During this minute you can think about anything you want except for a pink elephant. Whatever you do don't think about a pink elephant. Don't think about the elephant's big floppy ears. Don't think about the long trunk. Don't think about the massive feet. Don't think about hot pink elephants or lolly pink elephants or even elephants with pink polka dots. Got it? No pink elephants. Got it? No pink elephants . . .

Ready . . .

Steady . . .

Go!

So, did you accomplish it? My guess is that you thought of pink elephants. Sometimes people say that they managed to avoid thinking of pink elephants by deliberately thinking of something slightly different, like blue elephants. But really, is that helpful? Did you really want to waste a minute of your life filling your mind with blue elephants just to avoid a thought of a pink elephant? My guess is that once you got through the minute you were thinking of pink elephants anyway. How do I know this? Because one of the things that makes this task impossible is that there's only one way to know that you've succeeded, and that is to check. In other words, you need to ask something like, 'Did I do it? Did I manage to avoid thinking of pink elephants?' and there it is—a thought of a pink elephant.

When the task is about not thinking about pink elephants this can all seem rather silly and trivial. But what if the thought is about infertility or miscarriage or stillbirth? What if the thought is about failing as a mum, or experiencing a painful labour, or something horrible happening to your baby—what then? Sometimes we think that the best way of coping with these kinds of thoughts is to get rid of them. But, just like trying not to think about the pink elephant, trying not to think these kinds of thoughts, ultimately, doesn't work. In fact, you probably noticed that you thought more about pink elephants in that minute of trying not to think about pink elephants than you ever have in your life. In the same way, trying not to think scary, painful or sad thoughts can result in a rebound effect of thinking these thoughts more than ever before.

Further, in our attempts to stop thinking these thoughts we may become very busy filling our minds with all sorts of distractions to keep these thoughts out. This doesn't mean that it is wrong or unhelpful to ever use distraction. A little distraction for thoughts and situations that are temporary (such as distracting yourself during a quick medical procedure) does no harm. But it does mean that there's a real trap in trying to distract ourselves from bigger recurring thoughts. Just as distracting yourself from thoughts of a pink elephant required you to fill your mind with other thoughts such as of a blue elephant, distracting yourself from frightening, painful or sad thoughts requires you to fill up your mind with other thoughts. Distracting ourselves requires a lot of effort and mind space, and with all that effort and mind space being used to create distraction, there's less left for being the mum you want to be.

There's yet another trap to be wary of when we struggle with ourselves: struggling with our emotions can cause them to multiply. For example, we may start out feeling *sad* about some of the changes in our life that have happened in becoming a mum. Then, instead of letting this feeling be, we may decide that this feeling is wrong. We may think that we should feel only happiness about becoming a mum and try to eliminate this feeling of sadness. This may lead to *fear* that feeling sad makes us a bad mum. Of course, the thought of being a bad mum also makes us sad. Then, on top of that we are *angry* at ourselves for feeling sad and fearful and we begin to feel *anxious* about becoming a mum. So, what started out as a bit of sadness has quickly grown into a whole lot of sadness, fear, anger and anxiety. How much easier would it be to simply accept the original feeling of sadness as a part of our journey to motherhood?

THE STRUGGLE AND BECOMING A MUM

Take a moment now to relate this back to your own journey. Are there particular thoughts, feelings or memories that you struggle with in your transition to motherhood? Are there thoughts that you tend to fight (such as thoughts about being a bad mum, thoughts about your baby, thoughts about something bad happening) or feelings that you try to get rid of (for example sadness, fear, anger or anxiety)?

What are your thoughts, feelings and memories?

....

....

....

....

....

....

....

How do you struggle with your own thoughts, feelings or memories? Are there particular things that you do to try to get rid of unwanted thoughts feelings or memories? For example, do you distract yourself, use food for comfort, or avoid specific situations or thoughts?

....

....

....

....

....

....

....

Do these strategies work? Sometimes you'll find that some of the strategies do work some of the time, particularly in temporary situations. If so, make note of this. But also consider, do they work completely? Do they completely eliminate the thought, feeling or memory?

....

....

....

....

....

....

....

Do your strategies have a cost associated with them? For example, do the strategies require you to put in effort or mind space? Do they require money or time? Do they involve actions that aren't in line with your values? Is it easy to both fight your thoughts, feelings and memories *and* be the kind of mum that you want to be? What are the costs associated with the strategies that you use?

....

....

....

....

....

....

....

....

LETTING GO OF THE STRUGGLE

Struggling with our own thoughts, feelings and memories is like getting caught in a rip. When swimming in the ocean, if we find ourselves getting dragged out to sea our first instinct may be to fight against it. We can see the shore, where we want to be, rapidly disappearing and it is tempting to put all of our efforts into fighting the rip and swimming back to the beach. But, in fact, this is exactly what you shouldn't do. When caught in a rip the best thing to do is to swim sideways across it, allowing it to pull you along until the pull of the rip lessens and you are able to swim to shore. If you directly fight the rip you simply end up exhausted, and that is when you are at most risk of drowning. Likewise, if we directly fight our own feelings, thoughts and memories we are likely to end up exhausted with no energy, time or mind space left for what's truly important: living your values as a mother.

In other words, the temptation is to put the struggle at the centre of our lives. The temptation is to think that if we could just win the battle against our nasty thoughts, horrible feelings and bad memories then we'd be happy and we could live the life we want to live.

Notice whether you are having this battle in your transition to motherhood. Do you sometimes get caught up in thinking that you need to eliminate your sadness, fears, anger or anxiety in relation to becoming a mum? Does it sometimes seem as if it is important to eliminate all of your negative feelings and self-doubt in order to be the mum you want to be? In fact, this is an unwinnable battle because we cannot win a battle with ourselves. What if, instead of putting this struggle at the centre of our lives, we put our values at the centre of our lives? What if you were willing to experience both the joy and the pain as you journeyed towards being the mother you want to be?

In the following chapters we'll be exploring in detail exactly how you can begin to let go of the struggle with your own thoughts, feelings and memories, and this will include building concrete skills that will assist you in this task. For now, it is important that you can see that letting go of the struggle and making your values the centre of your life is the move that you want to make.

ONE WOMAN'S STORY

Reading Amanda's story may give you additional insight into coping with the emotional pain involved in becoming a mother.
Amanda is 18 weeks pregnant. This is her third pregnancy after the first two ended in miscarriages at seven and eight weeks respectively. Even though Amanda is now 18 weeks pregnant and her doctor has reassured her that there is no cause for concern, she frequently feels bursts of anxiety about her pregnancy and is haunted by thoughts of losing this baby.

Amanda has not shared her experiences of miscarriage with anyone but her husband Robert, as they decided to keep all pregnancies a secret until 12 weeks. When she confesses her fears of another miscarriage to Robert, he reassures her that this is 'irrational' and that she needs to 'stop thinking about it'. Amanda knows that he is trying to be supportive, but she finds that she simply can't stop thinking about it. The more she tries the stronger the thoughts seem to become, until she finds herself so consumed with anxiety and sadness that she cannot enjoy the pregnancy at all. She also finds herself trying to cope with the anxiety by binge eating, especially chocolate. Although this provides temporary relief, she knows it isn't ultimately solving the problem and she also feels guilty about eating so much chocolate during pregnancy. This makes her feel like even more of a failure as a mum.

When Amanda reads that emotional pain and joy are attached, this immediately makes sense to her. She finds it a relief to realise that she has been unable to eradicate her anxiety about losing her baby not because she isn't clever enough or because she isn't using the right strategies, but because that's just how the human mind works. Amanda decides to take a different approach and to stop struggling with her feelings. She finds that this brings up a lot of unresolved grief around her previous miscarriages, and she decides to share her experiences with her closest friends. When she does so, she discovers that one of her closest friends has also had a miscarriage, and together they have a good cry and a frank discussion about the experience.

Amanda decides that now she has stopped trying simply to get rid of her feelings and thoughts about her miscarriages she would like to do something special, as a mum, for her previous pregnancies. She decides to write a letter to her two 'angel babies' and to plant a tree in her back yard in honour of her first two pregnancies. She likes the fact that her next child will one day play under the very same tree.

After resigning the struggle with her own feelings and thoughts, Amanda finds that while she still has moments of sadness for her miscarriages, and moments of anxiety for her current pregnancy, she is now able to notice the joy as well. She also finds that she has more energy and space for doing what's really important: becoming the mum she wants to be.

MY UNIQUE ADVENTURE
These comments may help you to understand how the information in this chapter might relate to your unique experience.

Becoming a confident mum
May be relevant to women at any stage who are struggling to find confidence in their own mothering, coping with self-doubt or coping with criticism and advice from others.

Usually we think of confidence as thinking positive, affirming thoughts about ourselves. We can try to become confident by deliberately attacking any self-doubts, and end up locked in a struggle with ourselves. This struggle is, of course, a distraction from actually becoming the mum we want to be. But what if confidence wasn't about eliminating self-doubt? What if confidence meant such wide self-acceptance that you let yourself be, as you are, self-doubts and all? What if you—all of you, the doubts and nasty thoughts included—could together move towards being the mum that you want to be? Notice the ways that you struggle with your self-doubt. Is the struggle working? Notice times when you stop struggling with self-doubt. How are those times different?

Reversing the downward spiral
May be relevant to women with a history of depression, at risk of postnatal depression or experiencing postnatal depression.
It may seem like the best thing to do is to fight the depression head on. Often, however, this kind of a fight just feeds the depression. A way forward is to step away from the fight with depression and instead focus on building an enriching and rewarding life based on your values. When such a life is built, feelings of happiness and joy often gradually return.

Grief and loss
May be relevant to any woman experiencing a loss, whether it be an obvious loss such as miscarriage or stillbirth, or the loss of pre-motherhood life, difficulty conceiving, an unwanted birth experience or motherhood being different from expectations.
Grief is the perfect example of the fact that pain and joy in life are attached. It is not possible to open your heart to love without also opening your heart to the pain of grief associated with losing your loved one. The question is, will you keep your heart closed to both the love and the pain or will you fling your heart wide open, allowing in the love and the pain as well?

How do I survive this?
May be relevant to women experiencing emotional challenges, tough physical symptoms such as morning sickness, or birth.
Sometimes the battle to survive can become part of the problem. We may think that surviving means thinking or feeling a certain way, and we can become engrossed in a battle with ourselves in order to 'survive'. But what if survival instead meant allowing yourself to live through your own experience just as it is? Notice the ways in which you struggle with your thoughts

and feelings in order to 'survive'. Is this working? Notice times when you stop struggling. How are those times different?

Living with worry and anxiety
May be relevant to women with a history of anxiety, women struggling with anxiety or worries, or women with a specific worry about motherhood.

Sometimes we can handle feelings of anxiety by trying to avoid them. This can include avoiding the thing that we are anxious about. When what we are anxious about is a lion, then running away can be helpful. But if what we are anxious about is holding our newborn premature baby, then running away doesn't get us where we want to go. Feelings of anxiety often arise just when we are about to do something that really matters to us. So, in order to do the things that really matter, we often need to be willing to accept feelings of anxiety. Notice the times when you feel anxious. How does your anxiety relate to what matters to you? Do you 'run away' from the anxiety? When you do so, how does this affect your ability to do what matters to you?

PUTTING IT INTO PRACTICE
- ✩ Notice the ways that you struggle with your thoughts, feelings and memories. Does the struggle work? Does it bring you closer to being the mum you want to be?
- ✩ Experiment with letting go of the struggle. Are there times when you let go already? If so, how are the times when you let go of the struggle different from the times when you struggle? Does it feel different? Are you better able to be the mother you want to be? Do you have more energy for other things?
- ✩ Notice times when you put the struggle at the centre of your life and times when you put your values at the centre of your life. What is it like to act based on avoiding pain? What is it like to act based on your values? Which is more fulfilling?

3

Living with monsters

You stand at the door to your heart gazing at your baby, who is waiting for you on the doorstep. You want to gather your baby up in your arms, fling the door of your heart wide open and carry your baby deep inside. But you notice that your baby isn't the only one at the door. Along with your baby there are also monsters; ugly, frightening monsters lurking in the darkness. These monsters include nasty thoughts, horrible feelings and bad memories; some are old familiar faces and others are new terrors. You are confronted with this question: do you put your energy into fighting with the monsters and trying to keep them out, or do you fling the door to your heart wide open to let your baby in and accept that some of the monsters might sneak in too?

In the previous chapter we saw that suffering and joy are two sides of the same coin and that in order to become the mum we want to be we may need to let go of our struggle with pain. In this chapter we explore the concept of letting go of the struggle in more depth. By the end of this chapter you'll have a taste of what letting go is and, from this, in later chapters we'll build up the skills needed to put the concept fully into practice.

MEET THE MONSTERS

The best way to begin is to bring the monsters out of the darkness. Usually, these nasty thoughts, feelings and memories lurk in the background in your life and you may not consciously realise the effect that they have on you. When we take the time to meet the fiends in broad daylight and get to know their tricks, we may realise that they aren't as threatening as we had thought. So let's look at the monsters in the light and see if we can see them for what they really are.

I'm not a good enough mum monster

The *I'm not a good enough mum* monster is a particularly ugly one. It likes to spin stories, focusing on your faults and mistakes, and loves to compare you to other mums. When this demon spins stories it uses a few editing tricks to ensure that you always seem like a terrible mum. For example, it will edit out anything you've done well, leaving just your mistakes. It will also cheat when it compares you to others. For example, it might weave into its story how poorly you've adjusted to motherhood in comparison to your sister, leaving out the fact that your sister already has three children and that you are doing no worse than your best friend. During pregnancy this monster may delight in spinning panic-filled stories about how you are about to fail dramatically.

If this monster is hanging around, there is probably a cloud of sadness hanging around too. If you get caught in a struggle with this monster, you'll find yourself wasting a lot of time either moping about feeling sad and horrible or trying to convince yourself that you are a good mum after all. Both of these, of course, are a complete distraction from your baby.

I must be a perfect mum monster

This bogeyman may not look so ugly at first (it may even seem helpful), but it will really get under your skin. It is particularly fond of keeping a running commentary of everything that you should be doing and all the mistakes that you have made. It will regale you with a constant list of 'shoulds'. During pregnancy you will hear a lot about what you should be eating (for example, no chips ever), what you should be doing (hours of pregnancy yoga), what you should be buying (the Rolls Royce of prams) and how you should feel (blissfully happy, constantly). As a mum, the monster will tell you how you should be feeding baby (such as on an exact three-hour schedule), how you should be responding to your baby (immediately and with joy every time), how your baby should be sleeping (like a dream in her cot), how your baby should be developing and behaving (quiet and content all day long) and how you should feel about your baby (still blissfully happy, constantly).

When you do make a 'mistake' by doing something outside this list of shoulds, this monster likes to make a big song and dance about it, usually by beating you with a stick. This monster hangs out with guilt and anxiety. If you're struggling with this ogre, you'll probably find yourself rushing anxiously through a list of shoulds day after day instead of actually *enjoying* motherhood. You'll also find yourself doing what you 'should' be doing rather than what your baby is telling you he needs in that moment (or what you need in that moment).

There is an irony right in the heart of this monster. Imagine for a moment what it would be like to have a perfect mother. Imagine having a mother who always knew everything you needed and gave it to you immediately, who was never tired or cranky or stressed, who ran a house like clockwork, who never needed a break and who never made a mistake. With a perfect mum, how would you learn to accept imperfection in others, to wait, to self-soothe, to forgive, to consider others or to accept your own mistakes? The joke of this fiend is that a perfect mum is actually the *last* thing your baby needs.

It's all my fault monster

This gremlin can be a pal to the first two monsters and may make an appearance when they do. It will tell you that everything negative that is happening with your baby is your fault, from difficulty conceiving, to miscarriages, to complications in pregnancy, to feeding difficulties and sleeping problems. The monster won't wait for there to be any actual evidence to support this conclusion. However, even when you *are* contributing to the negative situation, getting caught up in a struggle with this bogeyman still isn't helpful because this monster is all about blame, not about helping you to change.

You will know that you have been caught by this monster because instead of putting your energies into making the most of the situation and changing what you can, you'll find yourself stuck in the blame game and dwelling on the past. If this monster is around, expect to feel really guilty.

Something horrible might happen monster

The *Something horrible might happen* monster chatters about the future and likes to spin stories about all the horrible things that might happen. Its big trick is to show you the terrible thing in horrific detail and then freeze-frame the situation right when it is at its absolute worst. For example, this monster will play for you a horrible show of what birth might be like and freeze it right at its most terrible point—when you are in the most pain, when you are the most exhausted, or maybe when you get whisked away for an emergency caesarean. It will neglect to show you what would happen next, however: the pain ending, you getting your baby and life moving on.

If this monster is around then anxiety is probably around too. If you get stuck with this gremlin you'll find yourself wasting time worrying about the future instead of enjoying what is happening here and now.

It shouldn't be like this monster

The *It shouldn't be like this* monster has an exact and detailed plan of what motherhood should be like and what your baby should be like. According to this monster, anything that doesn't fit with its strict plan is wrong. If you get caught up with this fiend, it will have you and your baby caught in a cycle of repeating actions that just aren't working for either of you. This monster will try to convince you to spend all of your energies desperately seeking a way to force your baby and yourself back on plan. This is, of course, a distraction from knowing your baby as she actually is and from enjoying your own, unique experience of motherhood.

If you find yourself living in crisis mode, thinking that motherhood will be enjoyable once you've found a solution to the current 'problem' (once baby is sleeping through the night, once breastfeeding is established, once baby is on solids, once baby learns to fall sleep by himself . . .), then check for this demon skulking in the shadows.

My baby is doing it deliberately monster

This monster will whisper to you that your baby's actions, whether it be crying, difficulty feeding or refusal to sleep, are deliberate and calculated attempts to drive you crazy. It will spin stories about your baby's motives, with complete disregard for the facts of infant development. If you buy into the stories this bogeyman tells you, you can expect to feel a lot of anger and frustration.

You can also get stuck fighting with this monster. It may seem like you have to eliminate this monster in order to be a good mum. If you do get stuck in this way, you can expect to feel guilt.

Irrespective of whether you are trapped into buying into this fiend's stories or fighting them, getting stuck with this monster is a distraction from figuring out what can be done to improve the situation.

Do you relate to any of these monsters? If so which ones?

. . . .

. . . .

. . . .

. . . .

. . . .

Do you have other monsters? If so how do they work?

....

....

....

....

....

....

SEEING THE MONSTERS IN BROAD DAYLIGHT

When your demons make an appearance in your everyday
life they probably seem ugly, frightening and threatening.
But often once we've had a good look at the monsters in the
light of day we realise that they aren't as threatening as they
seem. As we just saw, the bogeymen each have their own little
tricks to make themselves appear scarier than they really are.
Recognising these scams for what they are can be helpful and
can allow us to stop taking the monsters so seriously.

It is also important for us to realise that all of our monsters,
whether they are using these little tricks or not, are gaining
power over us by using one big trick. That trick is this: they
con us into thinking that they are a real threat. In fact, however, all of these monsters are simply collections of thoughts,
feelings and memories. A thought, a feeling or a memory, no
matter how dreadful or painful it is, cannot actually harm you.
It can hurt (a lot) but it cannot physically damage you or your
baby or destroy your life. (Don't just take my word for it; see
for yourself if this is true after the next exercise.) A thought,
a feeling or a memory cannot directly control what you do and
so cannot stop you from being the mum that you want to be.

Consider the *Something horrible might happen* monster. When we
get caught up with this gremlin we usually find ourselves experiencing a rush of anxiety. Our heart may race, our breathing
accelerates, our palms become sweaty—and yet the horrible

situation hasn't actually happened. When we look at our monsters in the daylight, they turn out to be nothing but smoke and mirrors.

WHERE DO MY MONSTERS COME FROM?

You may be able to recognise why you have the particular monsters that you have; why your mind chatters as it does. If this helps you to see the monsters for what they are, an illusion, then this is fantastic. If you haven't considered this before, it may be helpful to think about where your particular monsters come from.

Beware of becoming obsessed with searching for the origins of your demons though. It is important to realise that *all* humans have these monsters lurking. They aren't a sign of being a damaged human; they are just a part of being human.

LIVING WITH MONSTERS

What do you want your journey to motherhood to be about: keeping the monsters out of your heart or inviting your baby in? Learning to live with your own mind chatter is not about learning to live inside the world that your mind creates. It is about learning to live with your inner critic by recognising that that is all it is: an inner voice. A voice that is sometimes right, sometimes wrong, sometimes helpful, sometimes unhelpful. It is about bringing your monsters into the daylight and learning to live with them as they are: all makeup and special effects. And it is about learning to live with your thoughts, feelings and memories and recognising that they cannot harm you if you don't allow them too.

Learning to live with your self-talk means that you stop taking these voices seriously. Think of your inner critic as a radio playing in the background. You don't have to listen, engrossed, to the radio, believing everything it tells you, nor do you have to fight with it. You can just recognise that the radio is there and leave it to play in the background, focusing your attention instead on your life and your baby.

MONSTER RADIO

Spend a couple of minutes completing an activity that relates to becoming mum. You could be preparing something in the nursery, or reading about pregnancy, or even simply being with your baby. While you complete the activity, have the radio (tuned to a talk-back show) or the television on. (There's no need to *watch* the TV, we're just using it for the audio.)

First, try to accept as true everything that is being said. Aim to complete your activity while also taking the television or the radio show very seriously, drinking in every word. Pretend that you believe absolutely everything you hear and that the content of the television or radio show is of utmost importance to your life.

Next, try to fight with the television or the radio show. Pretend that it is vitally important that you prove the television or the radio wrong. For example, if the television show is science fiction, you may be shouting at the television that there's no such thing as space ships, or if the show is a drama perhaps you are arguing with the characters. It is helpful to actually argue out loud.

What is it like to relate to the television or the radio show in these ways? What happened to your ability to complete the activity that relates to becoming a mum?

....

....

....

....

....

....

Now approach the television or the radio in a different way. Leave it on in the background but don't attempt to become engrossed in the show or to agree with what is being said. There is also no reason to fight with it. Just let the television or radio play in the background, focusing instead on completing the activity relating to becoming a mum.

What is it like to relate to the television or radio show in this way? What happened to your ability to complete the activity relating to becoming a mum?

....

....

....

....

....

This time use a voice-recording device on a mobile phone, MP3 player or computer to create your own personal 'monster radio'. Record some of the thoughts and stories that your monsters whisper to you. Say them into the recorder in the same words that you hear in your mind. For example, one woman may record, 'You are so stupid. You are a hopeless mum. Oliver deserves better than you . . . '.

Now set yourself up to complete an activity that relates to becoming a mum again. This time complete the activity with your 'monster radio' on in the background. Just like with the television or radio, see what it is like to buy into your mind chatter, giving it your rapt attention. Next, see what it is like to fight with your monster radio.

What is it like to relate to your inner critic in these ways? What happened to your ability to complete the activity?

....

....

....

....

....

Next, approach your mind chatter in a different way. Let your monster radio play without becoming engrossed in it or fighting with it. Just allow it to play in the background while you focus on completing the activity. It probably felt natural and easy to do this with the television show or radio, but it may feel difficult with the monster radio. Give yourself time to practise until you get a taste of what it is like. You may like to try this with a television show or the radio again to help remind yourself how to do it. Remember that although you may not be used to treating your monsters this way, it is exactly the same skill: simply focus completely on your activity. See if you can be playful about this and let yourself let go of taking the monster radio seriously.

What is it like to relate to your monsters this way? What happened to your ability to complete the activity that relates to becoming a mum?

....

....

....

....

....

....

You probably found that the activity was easier to complete and more enjoyable when you stopped taking the monsters so seriously. When you were taking your monsters seriously you may have found that you were a slave to them. Once the seriousness was dispelled, however, you might have been able to recognise, as a direct experience, that in fact they have no control over what you do. Perhaps now it is clearer why the monsters can actually do you no harm. Being able to live with your monsters in this way allows you to regain control of your life and get on with being the mum that you want to be, regardless of what your demons have to say about it.

Now that you have a feel for what it means to live with your monsters, in the following chapters we'll develop some of the skills you need to do so in your daily life.

ONE WOMAN'S STORY

Reading how Laura learned to live with the I must be a perfect mum monster may help you understand how you can learn to live with your own monsters.

For Laura, the *I must be a perfect mum* monster is an old, familiar face. In one form or another, Laura has been struggling with perfectionism and anxiety for all of her life. While her perfectionist standards have brought her academic and career success, they have also made her life perpetually stressful, and whenever she makes a 'mistake' she is swamped with self-blame and guilt.

Laura initially approached her pregnancy with the same perfectionist standards. She decided that she would eliminate from her diet not just alcohol, soft cheeses and the other food it is usual to avoid during pregnancy but also all caffeine, junk food, sweet food and processed food. Whenever she gave into her cravings for hot chips, or soothed her morning sickness with soft drink, she felt racked with guilt. Laura had also decided that every day during her pregnancy she would take a walk for forty minutes after work. When she came home exhausted and collapsed onto the couch instead, she felt like a failure.

Laura was tortured by thoughts about how her imperfections meant that she wasn't giving her baby the best start in life. She had already begun to obsess about everything that she would do 'right' as a new mum. Her pregnancy had turned from a joyful time into an anxious list of 'shoulds' punctuated by moments of oppressive guilt, and she was frightened that her life as a new mum would be more of the same.

Laura also realised that she didn't want her new baby to learn to approach her life in the same way. She had tried to stop being such a perfectionist before by fighting it, but this had never worked. Laura would simply become perfectionistic about not being perfectionistic, and then it would become

just one more thing to feel guilty about. You can't stop yourself
from beating yourself with a stick with another stick. Laura
knew that she needed another way.

When Laura read about the I must be a perfect mum monster,
she experienced immediate recognition. She completed the monster radio activity. Laura recorded her monster's perfectionist spiel
and then spent a couple of minutes looking at nursery furniture
online with her very own monster radio playing in the background.
She found that if she accepted what her monster radio told her,
or fought with it, then she lost the ability to focus on and enjoy
looking at the nursery furniture. It took some practice to begin to
treat it like a radio playing in the background, and Laura found it
helpful to repeat the exercise several times by alternating between
listening to an actual radio in the background and listening to
her own monster radio. She found that when she started to take
her monster less seriously, she could keep her focus on the nursery furniture and enjoy the moment for what it was.

Laura started to recognise the I must be a perfect mum monster
for what it was, just a collection of thoughts and feelings. She
realised that she didn't need to escape the monster either by
completing its tyrannical list of shoulds or by fighting it into
silence. Rather, she could learn to recognise and accept it as
merely the chattering of her own mind, which couldn't harm
her. As Laura began to take the I must be a perfect mum monster less
seriously, she also began to base her actions on her values as a
mum rather than needing to complete a list of imperatives to sat-
isfy the monster, and at last she started to enjoy her pregnancy.

MY UNIQUE ADVENTURE

These comments may help you to understand how the information in this chapter might relate to your unique experience.

Becoming a confident mum

May be relevant to women at any stage who are struggling to
find confidence in their own mothering, coping with self-doubt
or coping with criticism and advice from others.

Take notice of your critical or self-doubting thoughts. Are the thoughts the grumbling of the *I'm not a good enough mum* monster or the *I must be a perfect mum* monster? Instead of struggling with these ogres and trying to prove them wrong, or listening to the monsters and taking their doubts seriously, can you notice them playing like a radio in the background? Experiment with treating your critical or self-doubting thoughts as a radio.

Reversing the downward spiral

May be relevant to women with a history of depression, at risk of postnatal depression or experiencing postnatal depression.

If you are experiencing depression, it is likely that the *I'm not a good enough mum* monster is hanging around. Experiment with not taking this monster so seriously. See if you can treat this monster like a radio playing in the background. What happens then?

Living with worry and anxiety

May be relevant to women with a history of anxiety, women struggling with anxiety or worries, or women with a specific worry about motherhood.

If anxiety is present then the *Something horrible might happen* monster may be present too. This monster delights in making gloomy predictions about the future. Are you able to stop taking its forecasts so seriously? This doesn't mean that you need to argue against its predictions or that you can't prepare for all possible future events. It just means that after the preparing is done you treat the doom-laden prophecies like a radio playing in the background. Instead of focusing on your monster radio, keep your focus on what you are doing in just this moment. How is this different?

Playing the blame game

May be relevant to women at any stage who are caught in the trap of blaming themselves, including where they genuinely have contributed to the situation.

Are you caught up in guilty self-talk about everything you have done wrong? The *It's all my fault* monster must be hanging around.

The really tricky thing about this monster is that even if you genuinely did contribute to the situation, continuing to take this gremlin seriously will not help. Self-recrimination focuses on the past, which cannot be changed. The *It's all my fault* monster will not help you to make the most of the situation as it is right now. Are you able to let this monster grumble to itself in the background while you get on with making the most of things as they now are?

PUTTING IT INTO PRACTICE

✰ Focusing on one of your monsters, write down the stories that it tells you on a piece of paper. Fold the piece of paper and label it with the monster's name. Now put the piece of paper in your pocket and carry it with you throughout your day. Every so often, take out the piece of paper and read it, then put it back into your pocket. Are you able to carry the monster with you without taking it seriously?

✰ Start to greet your monsters when they pipe up. For example, when the *I'm not a good enough mum* monster starts comparing you to others in your mother's group, say, 'Oh hello, *I'm not a good enough mum* monster, you're back again!'

✰ Practise relating to your demons like you would to a radio or a television that's playing in the background. There's no need to agree with what they are saying and no need to fight with them either. Can you let your monster radio play in the background?

4

Mindfulness

In the last chapter we saw how learning to live with our monsters involves not allowing ourselves to be distracted by their constant grumbling in the background. By keeping our attention in the here and now, we regain power over our lives. But staying present in the here and now has another benefit too. The present moment is where the true joy of life is.

The skill of being able to keep our attention in the here and now is called mindfulness. In this chapter the skill of mindfulness is introduced, and ways of practising mindfulness are explored—both formal, traditional mindfulness practice and also how to practise mindfulness in your everyday life. Mindfulness, or staying present in the here and now, has many benefits. Once the skill of mindfulness is learned it can be used to change our relationship to our thoughts and feelings, to become a more responsive mum and to build a stronger relationship with our baby. These applications of mindfulness will be explored in future chapters.

WHAT IS MINDFULNESS?

Mindfulness is the skill of being able to bring our attention to focus on what we want our attention to focus on, in the here and now, without judgment. That may sound very simple—and it *is* very simple—but it is amazing how difficult it is to actually do. We spend much of our lives not being very mindful at all. For much of our day we are on automatic pilot, habitually and mindlessly going through the motions of our life while we are living in our heads, caught up in our own mental chatter or our imaginings about the past or the future. The truly sad thing is that when we do this, we are missing out on our lives.

The good news, however, is that mindfulness is a skill, so the more we practise mindfulness the better we'll get at it. Mindfulness has been practised by many people over thousands of years. You may have practised it before if you have tried meditation or yoga. Mindfulness as it is presented in this chapter is a no-frills approach that maintains the principles of mindfulness practice. In essence, mindfulness, just like other skills such as riding a bike or baking a cake, can be taught, practised and improved upon. Recently, modern psychological science has demonstrated that living mindfully has benefits for psychological wellbeing. A regular mindfulness practice can improve emotional stability and help people coping with depression, anxiety disorders and stress.

In order to improve your ability to be mindful you do need to practise. In the same way that you can't learn to ride a bike simply from reading about it, you can't learn mindfulness simply from reading about it. You need to try it out for yourself.

The following exercises are suitable for women at all stages of the journey, whether you are trying to conceive, pregnant or a new mum.

A TASTE OF MINDFULNESS

The purpose of this exercise is to give you an experience of living mindfully. In order to complete this exercise you will need a small amount of food such as a single biscuit or cracker. If you are currently experiencing morning sickness then choose something that is least likely to make you queasy, and time the exercise for a better part of the day. It is perfectly possible to practise mindfulness when you are feeling nauseous, but if your morning sickness is particularly bad this probably isn't the best way to introduce the concept. If this is the case, skip this exercise for now.

A taste of mindfulness exercise

Sit in a quiet spot where you won't be interrupted, with the biscuit or cracker in your hand.

Just pause for a moment . . .

Look at what is in your hand.

Imagine you are an alien from another planet and you've never seen this object before.

Touch it gently with your fingers and notice the texture.

Allow yourself to notice its smell.

Let your eyes explore it fully, as if you'd never seen such a thing before.

If thoughts pop into your head like, 'This is a strange exercise' or 'I don't like this', acknowledge these thoughts and then bring your attention back to what is in your hand.

Now slowly bring the object towards your mouth, noticing any changes as you prepare to eat it.

Place it gently into your mouth, noticing how it is received.

When you are ready, very consciously take a bite.

Notice the taste . . .

Chew it slowly . . .

See if you can notice when you first feel ready to swallow.

Swallow slowly, following the sensations of swallowing, sensing the food moving down into your stomach.

Hopefully this exercise has given you a small taste of what living mindfully is like. How does eating mindfully compare to how you usually eat? Often when people try this exercise for the first time they find the experience of mindfully eating one cracker or biscuit very different from how they usually eat. It is common to find that you enjoyed the biscuit or cracker more than you usually would because you noticed subtleties of taste and texture that you usually miss. This is one of the advantages of living mindfully. If we stay in the present moment we are more likely to notice and truly experience the positive and rewarding aspects of our life.

My thoughts about *A taste of mindfulness*:

....

....

....

....

....

....

....

MINDFULNESS OF BREATHING

Mindfulness has been a part of spiritual traditions and practices for thousands of years, and during that time one of the most popular ways of practising mindfulness has been to practise mindfulness of breathing. This is the classic way of practising mindfulness, for the simple reason that our breathing is always available for us to be mindful of it. If we practise mindfulness by practising mindfulness of breathing then we become very skilful at using our breathing as an anchor to bring ourselves back to the here and now. This then becomes useful in our everyday life because our breathing is always there, ready for us to use as an anchor.

The following mindfulness of breathing exercise presents mindfulness of breathing practice in a formal, structured way. It is a good idea, in order to understand mindfulness fully, to try out this structured exercise. You may be interested in practising mindfulness regularly in this structured way (though you may not, or it may not be realistic for you right now). We will address finding a mindfulness practice that suits you later on in this chapter; for now, simply give this exercise a go.

When doing formal mindfulness practice, posture is important. You want to practise in a posture that helps you to be mindful so the posture should help you feel both relaxed and awake. In terms of physical posture I recommend either sitting cross-legged on the floor on a cushion, or sitting on a chair with both feet on the floor and legs uncrossed. Sometimes people feel that they should practise mindfulness cross-legged on the floor (or even in fancy postures such as the lotus position) and that practising on a chair is wrong. In reality, there is no advantage to sitting cross-legged on the floor over sitting on a chair, so you should do what is comfortable for you. Lying down is also an option, but this has the disadvantage of making it easy to fall asleep. If you experience discomfort or pain while practising the exercise sitting up, however, it is fine to try lying down. Ensure that you sit with a straight back (it will help you to stay awake more easily) but in a comfortable, relaxed posture, as this will help to settle agitated thoughts.

Your eyes can be open without focusing on anything in particular and resting slightly below eye level, or hooded (half open and half closed), or closed. The main advantage of keeping the eyes open is that it helps you to stay awake, whereas the main advantage of closing one's eyes is that it helps to minimise distractions. You should do whatever works best for you at the time, depending on how tired or agitated you are feeling. Some people find that they generally prefer one or the other, and this is fine.

Your hands should be placed on your knees/lower thighs, gently folded in your lap or by your side. Again, simply choose whichever is most comfortable. You may find it helpful to record the following instructions (perhaps on your phone, MP3 player or computer) and play them back the first few times that you practise. You may also need the instructions beside you as you practise, peeking at them every so often. This is fine at first, but aim to start practising the exercise independently as you get the idea.

Mindfulness of breathing exercise

Get into a comfortable sitting position, ensuring that you have a straight back but allowing yourself to have a relaxed, comfortable posture. Settle into it. If you want to close your eyes, close them now. If you keep them open, let them rest gently. Let your hands rest gently on your knees or in your lap.

Just settle into this ...

Allow your mind to settle into the here and now.

Notice, gently, what is happening in the here and now.

Notice the sensations in your body ...

The floor or chair supporting you ...

Areas of warmth or cool.

Settle, gently, into noticing your breathing.

Notice the rhythm of your breathing ...

The gentle in and out.

Bring your awareness to the sensations in your abdomen as you breathe.

Feel your abdomen inflate with every in-breath ...

And deflate with every out-breath ...

If you like, you can place your hand on your abdomen to help yourself notice this rise and fall.

When you are ready, remove your hand and keep noticing the rise and fall ...

The in and out.

Notice the short pause between each in breath and each out breath.

Allow your breathing to happen naturally.

Try to cultivate a sense of curiosity and adventure as if you are genuinely interested in exploring exactly what it feels like to breathe. Notice every breath ...

In and out ...

Allow your breathing to be your breathing.

From time to time you might notice that your mind has wandered. That's okay; it is what minds do. Gently bring your attention back to your breathing.

Try to bring a sense of kindness, of openness to your experience.

Allow yourself to gently open to the breathing that is ...

Let yourself rest in awareness of your breathing.
When you are ready to end the exercise, do so gently, bringing your awareness with you back into the room.

The purpose of this exercise isn't to breathe in any particular way; it is just to notice your breathing as it happens. You have been breathing all your life. Have you ever really noticed your breathing in this way before? You probably noticed that during the exercise your mind wandered. Perhaps you are surprised at how difficult it can be to keep your attention on your breathing. It is completely normal for our minds to wander during mindfulness exercises. The purpose of practising mindfulness is not to stop our minds from wandering. This is very difficult and will only leave you feeling frustrated. Rather, the purpose is to *notice* when your mind wanders and to gently bring your attention back to your breathing.

If you do begin practising mindfulness of breathing regularly you will notice that sometimes your mind wanders frequently and sometimes it wanders less. This is not better or worse. As long as you practise *noticing* when your mind is wandering, you are practising mindfulness. It can be tempting to judge yourself harshly or criticise yourself when you find that your mind has wandered. However, true mindfulness has a non-judgemental quality to it. So, when you notice that your mind has wandered, try to bring your attention back to your breathing in a gentle, kind way.

My thoughts on *Mindfulness of breathing*:

....
....
....
....
....
....
....

MINDFUL WALKING

Mindfulness of walking is another classic way of practising mind-fulness that has been practised for thousands of years. Some people find that it is easier to practise mindfulness of walking than mindfulness of breathing, so if you found mindfulness of breathing difficult then mindfulness of walking is good to try. People who enjoy practising mindfulness in lengthy sessions often combine mindfulness of breathing with mindfulness of walking practice to relieve the discomfort of sitting too long in one posture. Mindfulness of walking can easily be practised in your everyday life by turning a walk that you regularly do (such as walking to the bus stop, walking to your desk at work, walking to your letterbox) into a mindful walk. You can practise mind-fulness of walking in your own home or take a mindful walk in a more picturesque setting, such as a nearby park.

Mindful walking exercise

Start by standing with your feet parallel and slightly apart so that your feet sit comfortably under your hips. Keep your knees soft and unlocked so that they can gently flex as you walk. Let your arms hang loosely by your side or hold your hands together in front of your body. Let your eyes rest, gazing straight ahead.

Let your mind settle gently into the here and now.

Notice the floor or the ground under your feet ...

Notice the physical sensations of your contact with the ground.

Flex your knees slightly, transferring your weight to each foot, and notice the sensations.

When you are ready, transfer the weight of the body into the right foot, noticing the changing pattern of physical sensations in the legs and the feet as the right leg takes over the support of the rest of the body. Allow the left heel to rise slowly from the floor, noticing the sensa-tions in the calf muscles as you do so, and continue, allowing the whole of the left foot to lift gently until only the toes are in contact with the floor.

Staying aware of the physical sensations, slowly lift your left foot and move it forward, placing the heel on the floor.

Allow the rest of your left foot to make contact with the floor as you transfer the weight of the body onto the left leg.

With the weight transferred to the left leg, allow the right foot to lift. Move it slowly forward, being aware of the changing patterns of sensations in the foot as you do so.

Focus your attention on your right foot as the heel makes contact with the ground. Notice the transfer of your weight to the right foot.

Continue in this way ...

Slowly walking.

It is as if you've never walked before and you are really interested in experiencing what walking is like ...

Aware of the sensations in the bottom of your feet as they make contact with the ground ...

Aware of the sensations in the muscles of the legs.

Move slowly, allowing yourself time to notice each sensation.

Keep your gaze soft and directed in front of you.

Notice each transfer of weight ...

Each contact with the ground ...

Each movement of your muscles.

If your mind wanders, gently bring your awareness back to the sensations of walking.

Use the ground as an anchor ...

Let the ground reconnect you to the present moment.

When you are ready, you can gently walk a little faster ...

At an easy pace ...

Still noticing each sensation of walking ...

Still being mindful ...

Keeping a mindful awareness of each step.

When you are ready to end this exercise do so gently, bringing your increased awareness with you.

My thoughts on *Mindfulness of walking:*

....

....

....

....

....

....

....

DEVELOPING A REGULAR MINDFULNESS PRACTICE

Just like learning to play the piano or to dance the tango, becoming good at being mindful requires practice. If you are interested in mindfulness you might like to begin a regular, formal mindfulness practice. If you would like to do so, such as by practising mindfulness of breathing daily, start by practising for a shorter length of time (five to 10 minutes is usually long enough to begin with) and then increase your practice sessions from there as you wish. If you are practising mindfulness of breathing for 30 minutes or longer, consider breaking up your practice with a short mindfulness of walking practice to stop yourself from becoming sleepy or sore. Plan your mindfulness practice for a time of day when you are likely to be able to practise well. It is best if you are awake and relaxed. A popular time to practise is in the morning, but any time is fine, so pick what works for you.

Many people don't have the time or the energy to have a regular, formal mindfulness practice. Even if you are very interested in mindfulness and would like to practise it regularly with mindfulness of breathing, this may be impractical at present. Time and energy are both in short supply during pregnancy and the postpartum period, so we must be realistic! Just because you can't or don't want to sit cross-legged and practise mindfulness of breathing every morning doesn't mean that you can't practise mindfulness. Remember that the essence of mindfulness is keeping your attention in the here and now, without judgment. You can practise this at any time, with any activity. As we saw earlier, you can try turning a walk that you regularly take (such as walking to the shops) into a mindful walk. You can also try practising mindfulness of breathing during moments during the day when you need to wait (for example, while waiting in a queue). A particularly good time to practise mindfulness of breathing for a busy mum is during your baby's feeds. Why not make one of those feeds your mindfulness practice session each day?

Lastly, you can also bring mindfulness into any daily activity. Some activities that you can try doing mindfully include showering, brushing your teeth, eating, drinking, washing dishes or ironing. Practising mindfulness regularly in this way can be deeply enriching if you are very busy. When we perform a task mindfully we often notice the rewarding aspects of the task and can feel a sense of peace and stability that grounds us during a busy day. When performed mindfully, simple tasks can be turned into enjoyable and nourishing 'me' time. Mindfulness practice can then be used to turn small moments into time for yourself, or household tasks into time that is truly self-nurturing and enjoyable. This is definitely a positive thing for a busy mum!

Think about the best ways for you to practise mindfulness. Remember to make your goals for practising mindfulness realistic. Even practising for two minutes a day may be beneficial. Remember also that your mindfulness practice doesn't have to take up extra time. Consider making your mindfulness practice a task that you will be doing anyway, such as a walk, a household task, having a shower or one of your baby's feeds.

I am going to practise mindfulness by:

. . . .

. . . .

. . . .

. . . .

. . . .

. . . .

WAKING UP (MINDFULNESS IN EVERYDAY LIFE)

In addition to practising mindfulness to become better at being mindful, we also want to be able to become more mindful in our daily lives. The purpose of this exercise is to introduce a quick method for regaining mindfulness in everyday life. This exercise, once learned, can be done throughout your day whenever you feel the need to anchor yourself in the present.

Waking up exercise

First, notice your breathing …
Use your breathing as an anchor to the here and now.
Notice any physical sensations …
Any thoughts …
Any emotions.
Notice your experience right now, as it is.
Gently open yourself up to your experience.

You can use this exercise throughout your day to wake up whenever you feel yourself becoming entangled in your own thoughts and you want to get yourself out of your head and back into the world. Also simply try to notice the times during your day when you are mindful and the times when you are living in your head.

ONE WOMAN'S STORY

Reading Sakura's story may help you to see how to apply mindfulness in your life.

Sakura and her husband Hiroshi have been trying to conceive for the past 10 months. After years of ensuring that they don't fall pregnant, they are shocked to find that it isn't as easy as they thought. Sakura is worried that they may have left it too late. She discusses their situation with their family doctor, who advises a complete health overhaul while they organise fertility assessments and specialist referrals. The doctor advises that they should both stick to healthy eating, get regular, light exercise, limit stress and have regular sex during Sakura's fertile times in order to maximise their chances of conceiving.

Sakura knows that she is going to find these lifestyle changes challenging, especially the instruction to limit her stress levels. She finds the work politics in her job very stressful and often finds herself stewing over the latest saga during the evenings and on weekends. Sakura usually winds down by drinking a glass or two of wine in the evening and, on bad days, by treating herself to a big bowl of ice-cream as well. She also has an emergency stash of chocolate in her desk at work to get through the stressful work days. But now these two ways of coping with stress are banned in the name of getting healthy for fertility, and Sakura is feeling more stressed than ever as she finds herself fretting not just over her job but also worrying about her fertility and when she'll fall pregnant.

Sakura knows that she needs to find a completely new way of coping with stress, and so she decides to try practising mindfulness regularly. She begins by practising mindfulness of breathing for 10 minutes every morning and being mindful during a 20 minute walk in the evenings after work.

At first she finds practising mindfulness very difficult. She is shocked by how busy her mind is and how hard it is simply to be still and pay attention to her breathing for 10 minutes. It feels like she is constantly dragging her attention back to her breathing. She knows that this is normal, however, and so she persists.

At the end of the first week she begins to notice some changes. Although practising mindfulness of breathing seems just as hard as ever, she has noticed that she is brooding over work matters less in the evenings. She is finding it easier to keep her attention in the here and now in her everyday life, and when she needs a mindfulness boost, taking a moment to focus on her breathing really helps. The more that she practises mindfulness of breathing the easier it is to use her breathing as an anchor in her everyday life. As the weeks go by she finds that she is getting better and better at managing her stress, not by directly fighting it, but by learning to stay fully present and to live her life one moment at a time. In some ways the stress is still there—the tempest still rages on. However, Sakura feels like she's found herself a place of calm and stability within the storm.

MY UNIQUE ADVENTURE
These comments may help you to understand how the information in this chapter might relate to your own unique experiences.

Reversing the downward spiral
May be relevant to women with a history of depression, at risk of postnatal depression or experiencing postnatal depression.
A regular mindfulness practice can be a useful component in a plan to manage or prevent depression. Make a commitment to practise mindfulness regularly. Even five minutes of mindfulness of breathing practice may make a difference. If finding the time to practise is challenging, however, then practise mindfulness of a daily activity instead. You may find it particularly useful to practise mindfulness while doing an activity that you usually enjoy when you aren't depressed (even something simple like having a cup of tea). What do you notice?

How do I survive this?
May be relevant to women experiencing emotional challenges, tough physical symptoms such as morning sickness, or birth.
Developing a regular mindfulness practice can lead to an enhanced sense of emotional stability. This sense of stability or peacefulness then leads to resilience throughout the difficult times. Even five minutes of mindfulness of breathing practice each day may make a difference. If it is difficult to find the time to practise this, then practise mindfulness of a daily activity instead. Make a commitment to practise mindfulness regularly for several weeks. As the weeks pass, notice any changes. Are you developing a sense of stability or peacefulness?

Living with worry and anxiety

May be relevant to women with a history of anxiety, women strug-gling with anxiety or worries, or women with a specific worry about motherhood.

A regular mindfulness practice can be a useful component in a plan to manage anxiety. Make a commitment to practise mindfulness regularly. Try even five minutes of mindfulness of breathing practice and see if it makes a difference. If finding the time to practise is challenging, then practise mindfulness of a daily activity instead. As you continue to practise, what effects do you notice? Are you finding a stable centre inside the anxiety?

PUTTING IT INTO PRACTICE

- ✫ Try practising mindfulness of the breath every day, even if for only five minutes. If time is an issue, remember that mindfulness can be practised anywhere with any activity. Try practising mindfulness of breathing the next time you find yourself waiting or, if you are a new mum, during a feed.
- ✫ Pick a daily activity and do it mindfully. You might like to perform a household task mindfully, take a mindful walk or eat a meal mindfully. What is it like to live your life with mindfulness?

5

Mindful
mothering

Mindful mothering means that our attention is right where our baby is, in the here and now. When our awareness is grounded in the present with our baby, then it is easier to notice our baby's needs and to respond in a natural way. We are also more likely to notice the rewards of being a mum because they exist in the here and now too. In this chapter the concept of mindfulness is applied to mothering using specific exercises to help you to practise mindfulness of your baby. Being aware of your baby's needs and noticing the details of your baby's blossoming personality is vital to becoming both a responsive and a happy mum.

WHAT IS MINDFUL MOTHERING?
Mindful mothering is about deliberately increasing your awareness of your baby by practising the skill of mindfulness. It is about bringing your attention back to the here and now with your baby, as opposed to allowing yourself to become entangled in thoughts about the past or worries about the future (including thoughts and worries about baby). If you are psychologically present with your baby, rather than busy in your own head, then you are more likely to notice your baby's cues,

needs, feelings and patterns. This noticing is the first step to being a responsive mum.

Mindful mothering also provides a foundation for enjoying motherhood and for nurturing your bond with your baby. You may have noticed already from your mindfulness practice that when you perform a task with mindfulness, being fully present, you are more likely to notice the pleasant aspects of the task and to find the task rewarding. When you eat a biscuit mindfully, for example, you are more likely to really taste and enjoy the biscuit. In the same way, mindful mothering is about really noticing your baby just as she is in the present moment. Instead of becoming entangled in your thoughts about your baby or yourself as a mum, it is about just being present with your baby. In this state you are more likely to experience the joys and rewards associated with mothering. You are also more likely to notice the positive and unique qualities of your baby, as well as the way that she develops over time, and this will nurture the growing bond between yourself and your baby.

MINDFULNESS OF BABY DURING PREGNANCY

This mindfulness exercise is especially for being mindful of your baby during pregnancy. If you are still trying to conceive then put this exercise to the side for the time being. If you have already had your baby, then skip this exercise and practise the next one, mindfulness of your baby.

It is ideal to do this exercise at a time when your baby is active because you'll be able to enjoy noticing your baby's movements—although if you are doing the exercise and your baby isn't active, that is fine too. Whatever your baby does during the exercise, the purpose is to simply be mindful of your baby as he is.

Mindfulness of baby during pregnancy exercise

Get into a comfortable position.

Let your mind settle gently into the here and now.

Use your breathing as an anchor to connect to the present moment.

Place your hands on your belly and bring your attention to your pregnant belly.

Notice the weight of your baby inside you ...

Notice the feeling of carrying another, of carrying your child.

Notice what your baby is doing ...

Is your baby moving? If so, gently bring your attention to his movements, to his kicks and turns and rolls.

If your baby isn't moving, notice that he is quiet at the moment ... maybe he is sleeping.

You may find that thoughts arise, perhaps distracting thoughts about other things, or perhaps thoughts about your baby. Maybe you find that worried thoughts or guilty thoughts or sad thoughts arise about your pregnancy, your baby or birth. If so, gently let these thoughts go and bring your attention back to your baby as he is in this moment.

You may find that feelings of love arise, or you may not. Either way, this is fine. See if you can simply be with your baby as he is right now, without pressure on your baby or on yourself to be any particular way. As you breathe each breath in, feel your breathing gently swirl around your baby and caress him.

Notice that your body is protecting and caring for your baby as best it can.

Gently bring your awareness back again and again to your baby ...

When you are ready to end the exercise, do so gently, bringing your increased awareness of your baby with you into your everyday life ...

This exercise can be performed during pregnancy to begin to create the habit of being aware of your baby.

During this exercise you may find that feelings of love for your baby arise. If this happens, then you should feel free to enjoy and nourish your loving feelings. However, it is also equally okay if feelings of love don't arise. There can be a lot of pressure on a mum to bond quickly and easily with her baby. The first step to developing a positive relationship with your baby is to be able to be present with your baby in a gentle way, accepting your baby as he is and accepting yourself as you are in that moment. This includes accepting your current feelings about your pregnancy.

Learning to love your baby will be covered in more detail in future chapters, but for now, just know that whatever feelings and thoughts arise during this exercise are okay. The purpose isn't to feel or think anything in particular; it is simply to keep your awareness on your baby.

My thoughts on *Mindfulness of baby during pregnancy*:

....

....

....

....

....

....

MINDFULNESS OF BABY

This mindfulness exercise involves staying present with your baby and noticing your baby, as she is, in the here and now. If you are still trying to conceive or are pregnant then skip this exercise for now (if you are pregnant, continue to practise mindfulness of your baby as in the previous exercise).

The first time you try this exercise, you may like to do so at a time when your baby is asleep as you will probably find the exercise easier while she is sleeping. However, I would encourage you also to try the exercise when your baby is calm and awake as well as when your baby is unsettled and fussy. If you try this exercise when your baby is awake and you notice that she has a particular need (such as a nappy change), it is okay to respond immediately to that need, continuing to be mindful of your baby as you do so. It is also fine to interact with your baby if she initiates it—for example, if she begins to babble then feel free to talk back. If she is unsettled it is okay to use settling techniques. Remember that mindfulness of your baby is about enhancing your ability to respond to your baby's needs. The purpose, no matter how your baby is or whether or not you need to respond to her, is simply to keep your attention in the here and now and on your baby.

Mindfulness of baby exercise

Let your mind settle gently into the here and now.

Use your breathing as an anchor to connect to the present moment.

Bring your attention to focus on your baby.

Perhaps your baby is in your arms or maybe you are watching your baby in her cot or on a rug.

Slowly cast your eyes over your baby, noticing the details of her body ...

Noticing her toes, her legs, her arms and hands, her little fingers ...

Noticing her face and the details of her features.

Really pay attention to your baby, as if seeing her for the very first time.

If your baby is in your arms, notice the weight of your baby and the feeling of her against your skin.

If your baby is in her cot or on a rug, you might like to gently touch your baby, noticing how it feels to connect to her with touch.

You might like to smell your baby, noticing her unique baby smell.

Notice your baby's breathing, the gentle rhythm of your baby's in and out breaths.

You might like to gently place your hands on your baby's chest or back to really focus on the breathing.

You may find that thoughts arise—perhaps distracting thoughts about other things, or perhaps thoughts about your baby. Maybe you find that worried thoughts, or guilty thoughts or sad thoughts arise about your baby ...

If so, gently let these thoughts go and place your attention back to your baby as she is in this moment ...

You may find that feelings of love arise, or you may not. Either way, this is fine. See if you can simply be with your baby as she is right now, without pressure on your baby or on yourself to be any particular way. If your baby is awake, notice her reactions.

If your baby becomes unsettled or is fussy, it is okay to try to settle her. As you are settling her, try to stay aware of your baby, try to be genuinely open to her fussiness, try to really notice what she is like when she is fussing.

Gently bring your awareness back again and again to your baby ...
When you are ready to end the exercise, do so gently, bringing your
increased awareness of your baby with you into your everyday life ...

As with the mindfulness of pregnancy exercise, during this
exercise you may find that feelings of love for your baby arise.
If this happens, that is wonderful and you should go ahead
and enjoy them. However, it is also equally okay if feelings of
love don't arise. There can be a lot of pressure to bond quickly
and easily with your baby. The first step to developing a positive relationship with your baby is to be able to be present with
your baby in a gentle way, accepting your baby as she is and
accepting yourself as you are in that moment.

Learning to love your baby will be covered in more detail in
future chapters but for now, just know that whatever feelings
and thoughts arise during this exercise are okay. The purpose
isn't to feel or think anything in particular; it is simply to keep
your awareness on your baby. If you are able to be psychologically present with your baby as she is in the here and now, then
you are open to getting to know your baby better, to understanding her needs and to discovering her unique personality. This
will enable you to strengthen your relationship with your baby.

My thoughts on *Mindfulness of baby*:

....

....

....

....

....

....

....

....

WAKING UP TO BABY (MINDFULNESS OF BABY IN EVERYDAY LIFE)
We can also adapt our exercise for waking up in everyday life to include our baby. This adaptation is for new mums. If you are still pregnant or trying to conceive, then continue to practise the waking up in everyday life exercise found in the previous chapter. Adding baby to this exercise helps us to become more mindful of our baby in our daily life.

Waking up exercise
First, notice your breathing.
Use your breathing as an anchor to the here and now.
Notice any physical sensations ...
Any thoughts ... any emotions.
Now, connect with your baby.
Notice your baby as he is in the present moment.
Notice any cues ...
Any needs ... any feelings.
Notice your experience and your baby's experience right now, as it is.
Gently open yourself up to your experience and your baby ...

Throughout your day, if you find your attention wandering or your mind getting caught up in thoughts—even thoughts about your baby ('Why won't he nap in his cot? Other babies nap in their cot ... What's wrong with him? What's wrong with me?')—gently bring your attention back to your baby. This will give you an opportunity to notice the special, unique qualities of your baby as well as his current needs. Try bringing your attention back to your baby at different times of the day and when your baby is in different states: when he is sleeping; awake and playful; awake and calm; or unsettled.

What do you notice about your baby?

....

....

....

....

....

....

What do you notice about yourself as a mum?

....

....

....

....

....

....

....

....

Don't forget to try being mindful of your baby when your baby is unsettled. You can still try to comfort your baby as you normally would. Also, try to practise mindfulness and really notice your baby in his unsettled state. Try as best you can to stay present with your baby as he fusses and cries. (*Hint:* Imagine that you know, for certain, that your baby is going to continue to cry for another hour no matter what you do. Can you stay present with your baby for that hour? How can you and your baby ride the emotional storm together?) What do you notice?

ONE WOMAN'S STORY
Reading Erika's story will give you a glimpse into how mindful mothering can be beneficial.
Erika knew that she wanted to 'be there' for her baby Xavier. She was determined to learn to understand his cues and be a responsive, loving mum. Erika wanted baby Xavier to grow up

feeling secure, safe and loved. She also wanted to give herself the space to really enjoy mothering. Being a new mum was definitely exhausting and at times very stressful. But Erika knew that it was also a special time in her life that would end too quickly. She wanted to take the time to actually enjoy the experience.

When Erika read about the concept of mindful mothering, this seemed to be exactly what she wanted to do. Erika began by making time each day to practise being mindfully aware of baby Xavier, even if it was just for a minute. She'd pause in what she was doing and just notice him. She'd keep her attention on Xavier, noticing his expressions, noticing the little tufts of hair on his ears, noticing how his eyes were so much like her own and his face so like his dad's, noticing the way he would move and kick about, noticing the feeling of his skin against hers, noticing his baby smell.

After spending time practising being mindful of baby Xavier, Erika would feel more connected to him. Sometimes thoughts would pop into her mind while she was paying attention to Xavier, usually thoughts about things that she needed to do during the day such as put a load of washing on, or make that appointment with her doctor. Sometimes the thoughts would be worried thoughts about whether she was a good enough mum. Erika found it both fascinating and ironic that her anxious thoughts about being a good enough mum could themselves get in the way of her becoming the mum she wanted to be. Erika would let go of these thoughts and bring her attention back to just noticing baby Xavier.

Erika found that the more she practised being mindful of Xavier, the more she could keep her attention in the here and now with him during the day. She discovered that if her attention was in the here and now with her baby, she was more likely to notice the cuteness of his smile or the cleverness of his babbling. Erika found she was able to enjoy the rewards of being a new mum more because her attention was in the here and now to notice them.

Erika also realised that if her attention was in the here and now with Xavier, she was more likely to notice her baby's cues, needs, feelings and patterns. The more aware she was of baby Xavier's cues, feelings and needs, the better she could respond. Of course, there were still stressful moments, but Erika found that mindful mothering could be useful in times of stress too. When baby Xavier was grizzly, for example, Erika had a tendency to become lost in her own worries about him ('Is he sick? Is this normal? Why does he fuss so much? Am I doing something wrong?'). By bringing her attention away from her own thoughts and focusing instead on her baby in the present moment, Erika had more success at reading Xavier's cues and being persistent in trying strategies to settle him. Erika was able to truly 'be there' for her baby.

MY UNIQUE ADVENTURE

These comments may help you to understand how the information in this chapter might relate to your own unique experiences.

Becoming a confident mum

May be relevant to women at any stage who are struggling to find confidence in their own mothering, coping with self-doubt or coping with criticism and advice from others.

If you are able to stay psychologically present with your baby, then you have taken a big step towards finding your feet as a mum. Finding your own mothering style, and being confident in it, is easier the better you know your baby. The more you notice your baby as she is in the here and now, the more you'll see her unique cues, needs, feelings and patterns.

Being a mindful mum takes practice, so commit to practising staying present with your baby regularly, even if it is just for five minutes a day. Also, as best you can, bring your attention back to your baby, as she is in the here and now, regularly throughout your day. With practice, do you find yourself getting to know your baby's cues, needs, feelings and patterns?

Becoming Mum ... again

May be relevant to women with older children who are pregnant or have a new baby

Mindful mothering can be used with older children too. Spending time together, mindfully, can be a wonderful way to connect to them and show them love. This is helpful when you are coping with the challenges of pregnancy or a newborn baby and they are coping with a new sibling. Choose a daily activity that you do with your child (such as giving your child a bath, eating together, reading your child a story, breastfeeding, cuddling to sleep) and ensure that you do that activity mindfully, paying full attention to your child and noticing the unique individual that he is. What did you learn about your child? What is it like to be with him, enjoying him as he is?

Reversing the downward spiral

May be relevant to women with a history of depression, at risk of postnatal depression or experiencing postnatal depression.

When we are depressed we stop noticing the joys and rewards in our everyday life, and this makes the depression worse. By bringing our attention back to the here and now with our baby, we can begin to notice the rewards that being a new mum can bring, and so break the cycle of depression.

Start practising mindfulness of your baby regularly, even if it is just for five minutes. Remember that you can practise mindfulness while you are performing another activity such as feeding your baby, bathing your baby or playing with your baby. When you perform these activities with mindfulness, what do you notice about your baby? If there are specific activities that you enjoy or activities that you expected to enjoy with your baby, then practise these with mindfulness. It may take time for the glimmers of joy to appear, so make a commitment to practise for several weeks. As you continue practising, do moments of joy with your baby begin to appear?

Living with worry and anxiety

May be relevant to women with a history of anxiety, women struggling with anxiety or worries, or women with a specific worry about motherhood.

If you are feeling a lot of anxiety, then you may be spending time caught up in thoughts about the future. The trouble is that your baby exists in the here and now. Mindful mothering is about bringing your focus back to the here and now so that you can be with your baby. This takes practice. Practise bringing your attention back to the present with your baby, even if for only five minutes a day. Also, as best you can, bring your attention back to your baby as she is in the here and now regularly during your day. Does this lead to better connection with your baby?

PUTTING IT INTO PRACTICE

☆ If you are pregnant or a new mum, set aside some time to practise mindfulness of your baby, even if it is just for five minutes. During this time, keep bringing your attention back to your baby as she is. What did you notice about your baby? Make a commitment to practising mindfulness of your baby regularly. After several weeks of practising, what have you noticed? Are you better at staying in the present moment with your baby? Does this make a difference?

☆ If you are pregnant or a new mum, try to build a habit of being mindful with your baby in your everyday life. As best you can, stay present with your baby as she is in the here and now. What do you notice about your baby? If you are a new mum, pay attention to your baby's cues, signs, feelings and patterns. What have you learnt about your baby? Has this changed how you respond to your baby?

☆ At times, as a new mum, your own thoughts—even thoughts about the baby—might get in between you and your baby. For example, you may find yourself distracted by anxious thoughts about your baby's future. Notice the times when this happens, and try as best you can to bring your attention back to the present moment with your baby as she is, in the here and now.

6

Thoughts are just thoughts

Normally, we take our thoughts very seriously indeed. Have you ever found yourself lost in your thoughts, having a detailed imaginary conversation with someone or experiencing in vivid detail a potential future event? Have you found yourself actually becoming anxious or angry or sad? It is easy to get caught up in our thoughts and react to them as if they were real. It can be helpful to remember that our thoughts are just that—thoughts.

In this chapter we will explore thoughts in greater depth and build the skills needed to relate to thoughts as thoughts. In doing so, we will draw upon the concept of mindfulness again and learn how to be mindful of our thoughts. Getting some breathing space from our thoughts allows us to live in our life and not in our head.

GETTING CAUGHT IN OUR THOUGHTS
Imagine for a moment your favourite food. Let yourself think about the smell of the food and what it looks like. Imagine taking a bite, think about the taste of it on your tongue and the feel of it in your mouth. Now, notice your reactions. Are you getting hungry? Salivating? Feeling ready to eat? You've probably noticed that you've begun to respond emotionally and

physically to the food. Yet there is no food present. This is kind of strange, isn't it? Why do you have this reaction?

You have this reaction because we humans naturally respond to our thoughts as if they are real. This ability allows us to problem solve by imagining a potential situation, feeling our reactions to it and thinking through our best options in that situation. For example, during pregnancy you might think to yourself (as many women do), 'What if I have to have an emergency caesarean?' You can imagine in detail what that might involve, how it may occur, what the midwives or the doctors might say. Once you begin to think about having an emergency caesarean, you'll start to respond emotionally as if it is actually happening. In other words, you may start to feel anxious or sad or relieved, as if you are really there having the caesarean. And now that you have a taste of what your reactions may be in the situation, you can plan accordingly. Maybe you'll plan for an extra support person to be rung, or for your partner to be the one to present your baby to you if you have to have a general anaesthetic.

Being able to imagine our reactions in novel situations and create these plans is very useful. However, we are so good at responding to our thoughts as if they are real that we often get caught in them. We get stuck living in our head rather than living our life. In this way, even after fully thinking through the situation of having an emergency caesarean and creating a plan, a woman may continue to be caught up in her thoughts about emergency caesareans, continuing to respond emotionally as if it is actually happening. She may continue putting herself through the emotional experience of having an emergency caesarean over and over throughout her pregnancy. Each time she imagines it she responds as if it is real, feeling all the anxiety she'd feel knowing that she has to have it and all the sadness of missing out on a vaginal birth. How exhausting!

Of course, we can also experience a similar problem in getting caught up in our memories. In this way, a woman who has actually had an emergency caesarean may continue to replay the memory of the procedure in her head, getting caught up in the memory and continuing to respond emotionally as if it was still happening. It is as if she didn't just have one caesarean but many, as she relives the experience again and again.

Either way, if a woman is stuck in her head worrying about a caesarean while she is pregnant, or remembering the caesarean as a new mum, she isn't fully living out the joys of the here and now, enjoying her pregnancy or her baby.

In terms of our thoughts, we also have to contend with the whisperings of our monsters. Many of these thoughts can be bullying. We may experience thoughts like, 'I am stupid', 'I am a hopeless mum' or 'I can't cope'. Imagine that a real person was in your home following you around and whispering into your ear the kinds of bullying thoughts that you have from time to time. If you had a real person whispering these things to you, would it be surprising to find that you feel sad or anxious? Yet, because we naturally respond to our thoughts as if they are real and because we tend to get caught up in our thoughts, we may very well respond emotionally to them as if they were the taunts of a real bully.

It is important to emphasise that this isn't about whether your thoughts are true or false. The thought, 'childbirth will be painful' is true for most women. Even if you end up experiencing no pain in childbirth (wow, lucky you!), it is still helpful to have this thought during pregnancy and to act on it by seeking information on your pain management options so that you can decide what is right for you. However, beyond this practical response, it is not useful to dwell on this thought. Even though it will likely prove true for you, it is not helpful to spend your pregnancy imagining the pain of childbirth, responding emotionally as if you are experiencing that pain again and again. It is enough to experience the pain of childbirth when you are actually experiencing the pain of childbirth. There is no benefit to trying to cope with it throughout the whole pregnancy as well.

Therefore, it is irrelevant whether our thoughts turn out to be true or false, there is no need to argue with them or to find out which are correct. And in that case, what *do* we need to do then? The answer is that we need to build the skill of relating to our thoughts mindfully. This means that we are aware of our thoughts merely as thoughts, and we are able to let go of even sticky thoughts, to disentangle ourselves from them, and return our attention to the here and now of our lives.

MINDFULNESS OF THOUGHTS

We can use our mindfulness skills to practise mindfulness of our thoughts themselves. Being mindful of our thoughts is about focusing our attention on our thoughts without getting caught up with them. In other words, it is about noticing them and being aware that they are just thoughts rather than responding to them as if they are real.

The following exercise can be used to build the skill of being mindful of your thoughts. It involves visual imagery and thus it is best done with your eyes closed. This exercise is suitable for women at all stages, whether you are pregnant, a new mum or trying to conceive.

Mindfulness of thoughts exercise

Get into a comfortable sitting position, ensuring that you have a straight back but allowing yourself to have a relaxed, comfortable posture. Settle into it. For this exercise, gently close your eyes. Let your hands rest gently on your knees or in your lap.

Allow your mind to settle gently into the here and now.

Notice the sensations in your body . . .

Feelings of touch or pressure where your body makes contact with the floor or the chair . . .

Feelings of warmth or cool . . .

The rhythm of your breathing . . . the gentle in and out.

Notice the sensations as you breathe.

Use your breath as an anchor to connect to the here and now.

Bring your awareness to the thoughts that arise in your mind.

As best you can, try to watch your thoughts come and go.

You may like to imagine that you are sitting next to a stream and that the stream is your mind ...

Your thoughts are like leaves on the stream ...

Every so often you notice a thought arise; that thought flows through your mind for a while and then disappears again.

You might notice that some thoughts keep coming back. That's okay. Just keep noticing the thought as a leaf on the stream ...

Notice that the thought arises, flows through your mind for a while, then disappears again.

You might also find that you have thoughts about this exercise, maybe thoughts like, 'This is boring' or 'This is difficult'. Just notice that these thoughts, too, are thoughts.

Stay watching your thoughts as best you can ...

Every so often you might get sucked into your thoughts and find that the thoughts carry you away. If this happens, that is okay. Congratulate yourself on becoming aware of this even if it happens repeatedly, and pull yourself out of your thoughts and back to watching them.

Perhaps you aren't finding the image of a stream helpful. You can try other images, like clouds in the sky or a TV screen, or even no visual image at all. What is important is that you are watching your thoughts. Notice the thoughts arise then fade away ...

Notice your thoughts, coming and going, and notice that you are watching them.

If you find yourself being dragged away by your thoughts, dragged into a remembered past or a hypothetical future, then gently pull yourself back to watching the thoughts come and go.

When you are ready to finish, do so gently, using your breathing as an anchor to bring your awareness with you back into the room ...

This exercise uses visual imagery to help you to focus on your thoughts and to notice them as thoughts. Many people find the visual imagery useful, and you can experiment with different images to find what works best for you. It is important to note, however, that the imagery itself is not important. Some people find visual imagery difficult to create or unhelpful. If this is the case, you don't need to use any visual imagery at all. What is important is that you spend time watching your thoughts and watching them come and go. If you like, you can practise mindfulness of thoughts as a set exercise regularly in order to improve your ability to be mindful of your thoughts as thoughts.

My thoughts on *Mindfulness of thoughts*:

....

....

....

....

....

....

NOTICING THOUGHTS AS THOUGHTS IN EVERYDAY LIFE

When practised regularly, the *Mindfulness of thoughts* exercise can improve your ability to be mindful of your thoughts. However, we also need some quick and easy techniques to remind ourselves during our everyday lives that our thoughts are just thoughts. These techniques can help us detangle from our thoughts so that we stop reacting to them as if they were real and begin reacting to them as they are, as mere thoughts. There are no set strategies for doing this that work for everyone. If you try out some of the techniques described below, you will find that some work well for you and others not so well, so find the ones that work well for you and use these. All of these techniques are suitable for women at all stages, whether you are pregnant, a new mum or trying to conceive.

In order to try out some of the following techniques, you will need to start by getting yourself tangled up in a thought. First, we'll try some techniques for detangling you from verbal thoughts. So begin by thinking of a nasty bullying thought that is particularly sticky for you—perhaps, 'I'm a bad mum'. Think it through a few times and let it entangle you. Then try out the strategies below. In between trying the various techniques, allow yourself to really buy into the thought again. See which of these techniques work for you in helping you to detach yourself from the thought. Try:

- ✩ singing the thought aloud—maybe to a well-known tune, such as 'Happy birthday'. For example, you might be singing out loud, 'I'm a bad mum, I'm a bad mum, I'm a bad mum' to the tune of 'Happy birthday'
- ✩ saying the thought in a funny voice—for example, you might be saying the thought, 'I'm a bad mum' out loud in the voice of a cartoon character
- ✩ prefacing the thought with, 'I'm noticing that I'm having the thought that . . . ', for example, instead of saying, 'I'm a bad mum', you might say, 'I'm noticing that I'm having the thought that I'm a bad mum'
- ✩ relating to your thought as a separate character and thanking it—you could call this separate character 'Mind', or even call it after the monster that this thought relates to. For example, after thinking, 'I'm a bad mum', you might say, 'Hi, *I'm not a good enough mum* monster. Thanks for pointing that out'.
- ✩ picture the thought as a leaf flowing down the stream—this works best if you practise mindfulness of thoughts regularly.

Some of these techniques may have worked better than others. Note down which techniques you found most effective:

....

....

....

....

....

....

Many troubling thoughts aren't verbal. They may be more like movies playing in our head. We often replay bad experiences from the past in our mind or play scary future scenarios.

For example, during pregnancy, many women may play in their mind their most feared future birth experience. Again, you need to try out the techniques and find which works best for you. The first step is to bring to mind a scenario that plays in your head, either a frightening future scenario or an experience from the past. Take a moment to really delve into the experience and become ensnared in it. See which of these techniques work for you in helping you to detangle from the thought. Try:

✮ putting the scene onto a television or a movie screen and stepping back from the screen, perhaps even experimenting with pressing buttons like Pause or Rewind, or seeing yourself eating popcorn as you watch (So, if you are getting stuck in imagining yourself giving birth, see the birth unfolding on a television screen while you watch it, eating popcorn.)

✮ putting the scene onto a computer screen and finding yourself sitting at the computer, perhaps playing and pausing the images like a movie or YouTube clip (See the birth unfolding as a YouTube clip while you sit at the computer.)

✮ freezing the scene right when the scenario is at its worst, and envisaging it as a painting. Put a large frame around it and hang the painting on the wall. (See the birth as if it were a painting on your wall.)

Again, some techniques probably worked better than others for you. Which techniques were most effective?

....

....

....

....

....

....

Of course, you may also create your own strategies. This is wonderful, and you should feel free to have fun experimenting with relating to your thoughts as thoughts. Remember that the purpose is to jolt yourself out of reacting to your thoughts as if they were real and to instead react to them as they are, as thoughts. Being able to relate to your thoughts in this way puts you in control of your life, so that you are able to live in your life rather than in your head.

ONE WOMAN'S STORY
Reading Melanie's story may help you to see how to relate to your thoughts as thoughts.

Melanie went to her 20 week ultrasound full of excitement and anticipation. She was thrilled to be getting a glimpse of her baby. As Melanie is a single mother, her main support person is her own mum, Vanessa, so she invited her mum along to the big event. They both delighted in watching Melanie's baby on the screen and were excited to find out that the baby was a boy.

Melanie also took her mum to her obstetrician appointment the next day to discuss the scan. The obstetrician explained that the ultrasound had revealed a cyst on her baby's brain but that this should be considered a normal finding at this stage because there were no other causes for concern. He stated that many babies have cysts at 20 weeks that disappear as they continue to grow, and suggested that they repeat the ultrasound in the third trimester. The obstetrician assured Melanie that there was no reason for her to worry. Melanie was glad that she had her mum with her because she left the obstetrician's office in a panic. Although she understood that her baby was probably completely healthy and that the cyst wasn't a concern, it hadn't truly occurred to her before that day that her baby might not be 100 per cent healthy. She began to worry.

Melanie found herself brooding over concerns about her baby's health. She would wake up at 2 am with her mind filled with visions of every disability or medical complication that her little baby boy could be born with. She would imagine each scenario in vivid detail, feeling sick with worry as she did so.

Melanie wished that she could somehow check on her baby and know that he was completely healthy. She began to long to get through the pregnancy to the birth so that she could see for herself that her son was okay.

When she shared this feeling with her mum, Vanessa shook her head and said that Melanie needed to learn to live with the worry. She explained that she still had worrisome thoughts about Melanie's health, and that just as Melanie had thoughts about the medical complications her baby might have, Vanessa had thoughts about the medical complications that Melanie could have in pregnancy or during childbirth. Melanie realised that her anxious thoughts were a normal part of becoming a mum, and that while they were useful in preparing her for all eventualities, the trouble was that she was getting stuck in them. She knew that she needed to learn to live with her thoughts without dwelling on them.

Melanie recognised that her worrisome thoughts were just that—thoughts. It wasn't helpful for her to continue to respond to them as if they were real. Although it was natural for her to have the anxious thoughts, she needed to be able to disentangle herself from them.

Melanie began to practise mindfulness of thoughts by imagining her thoughts as leaves on a stream for five minutes every morning. She also began to detach herself from her imaginings of her baby having a disability or medical complication by imagining seeing the images on a television screen. Watching the scenario unfold on a television screen in her imagination gave Melanie some distance from it. This reminded her that her thoughts were just thoughts. Once disentangled from her thoughts she could reconnect to where she was in the here and now and continue to enjoy her pregnancy.

MY UNIQUE ADVENTURE
These comments may help you to understand how the information in this chapter might relate to your own unique experiences.

Becoming a confident mum

May be relevant to women at any stage who are struggling to find confidence in their own mothering, coping with self-doubt or coping with criticism and advice from others.

The techniques described in this chapter are ideal for extricating yourself from self-doubting and critical thoughts. In the past you may have tried to become confident by fighting such thoughts, but what if instead you simply detached yourself from them and were able to see them as they are—mere thoughts? Experiment with the techniques for getting unstuck from your thoughts and find which works best for you. Try them out in your everyday life.

How do I survive this?

May be relevant to women experiencing emotional challenges, tough physical symptoms such as morning sickness, or birth.

Often when the here and now is at its most difficult and most painful, we make things worse again by dwelling on how bad things are. Sometimes we try to counteract this by struggling with our thoughts, maybe even trying to force ourselves to think that things are wonderful. What if instead we could learn to see our thoughts as just thoughts? Find the detangling techniques that work best for you and try them out in your life. Does becoming disentangled from your thoughts help you to remove that extra layer of pain that is added by thoughts?

Living with worry and anxiety

May be relevant to women with a history of anxiety, women struggling with anxiety or worries, or women with a specific worry about motherhood.

Often when we are anxious we are living, in our mind, a potential future scenario in which everything is going wrong. We can become so caught up in this imaginary future that even after we've taken all useful steps to prevent or prepare for the situation that we envisage, we can continue to live and relive the imaginary situation in our heads. We can become so trapped that we believe the only way to cope is to come up with an answer to these thoughts and prove them wrong, and so we may find ourselves worrying, thinking over the statistics, the possibilities, everything that we can do. However, we can never perfectly control the future, and so the anxiety and the worry continue.

But what if instead we could live with these thoughts about the future as they are; just thoughts? What if we could bring ourselves back into the here and now? The next time an imaginary future scenario carries you away with anxiety, try out the strategies for getting unstuck from your thoughts. Are you able to disentangle yourself from the imaginary future scenario and bring your attention back to the present moment?

PUTTING IT INTO PRACTICE

☆ Do you find yourself getting caught up in your own thoughts frequently? Do you find that your thoughts come between you and your baby or between you and becoming the mum you want to be? If so, you can try practising mindfulness of thoughts regularly by imagining your thoughts as leaves on a stream (or using another visualisation that you find helpful). With regular practice you will find that you get better at noticing your thoughts as thoughts.

☆ Experiment with the different techniques for getting unstuck from your thoughts. Which strategies do you find most helpful?

☆ Try using the detangling techniques in your everyday life whenever you find yourself trapped by your thoughts. Does it help you to remember that your thoughts are just thoughts? Do you find that you are then more present in your life?

7

The emotional journey

The journey to motherhood is an emotional roller-coaster. From trying to conceive, through pregnancy and into motherhood, there are emotional highs and lows, often experienced through a haze of exhaustion. Like many women, you may find that throughout the transition you experience the greatest emotional highs of your life, along with the deepest lows. When we lack awareness of our emotions, or we cannot allow our emotions to be as they are, our emotions gain control of our actions. We may act on automatic pilot, allowing emotions to determine what we do, or we may choose our actions in order to try to eliminate specific emotions. However, if we are aware of the emotional aspects of our voyage and accept our emotions for what they are, a natural and healthy part of becoming a mother, then we maintain power over our lives.

In this chapter we'll explore emotions and build skills of awareness and acceptance of emotions, drawing upon the skill of mindfulness outlined in the previous chapters. If we can be aware and accepting of our emotions then we gain control of our life, freeing us to become the mum we want to be.

MINDFULNESS OF EMOTIONS

When we lack mindfulness of our emotions, our emotions are in control. We function on autopilot, slaves to our emotional reactions. We may not even be aware of smaller emotional fluctuations, and then when bigger emotions surface, they may take us by surprise and we may find ourselves swept away by the force of our feelings. When this happens, we may find ourselves doing or saying things that are completely against our values, things we never wanted to do or say.

Mindfulness of emotions goes hand in hand with acceptance of emotions. Often when we lack awareness of our emotions we also lack acceptance of them. We may think things like 'a mother should never feel angry with her child' or 'a mother should feel love for her baby from birth'. When we are unaccepting of our emotions as they actually are, then we may not be in touch with the smaller waves of emotion, and then when the big wave comes we may be unprepared for it. For example, imagine a breastfeeding mum experiencing a feeding frenzy as her baby feeds every hour into the night to boost milk supply. If the mother isn't mindful or accepting of her emotions, then when she is woken again at 3 am after being woken every hour all night, she is vulnerable to being overwhelmed by the wave of anger that she may experience, and to acting on it. However, if she is mindful and accepting of her emotions then she will have already noticed that her feelings of frustration are building, she will have accepted that feeling angry in such a situation is normal, and she is more likely to notice the big wave of anger approaching. This means that she can draw on coping strategies and supports to ensure that she isn't overwhelmed by her feelings of anger; for example, by waking her partner, putting on some music or phoning a helpline.

We can also find ourselves making bargains with our emotions, bargains intended to avoid or block out our

feelings, often at a cost to our values. We may find ourselves using alcohol, drugs, distraction, keeping busy, food
or even simply avoiding the situation or people altogether
in an attempt to dodge our emotional experiences. In small
doses, used from time to time, many of these avoidance
strategies aren't problematic. However, when we use these
avoidance strategies frequently to block out our emotions,
they can do long-term damage to our physical and mental
wellbeing, and prevent us from living our values.

Finally, remember what we learnt in the second chapter
about joy and pain? If we don't accept our emotional experiences as they are—if we try to fight them—usually the
emotions only multiply. So the woman experiencing anger
at her baby at 3 am who isn't accepting of her emotions may
end up also feeling guilty and sad and angry at herself. And
how does any of that help the baby?

Fortunately, we can, with practice, become increasingly
mindful and accepting of our emotions. The following
exercise involves practising approaching emotions with
awareness and acceptance. This exercise uses visual imagery,
so it is best done with your eyes closed. Like the mindfulness
of thoughts exercise, most people find the visual imagery
helpful, but if you don't it is okay to practise increasing your
acceptance of your emotions without the imagery.

The first time you try the exercise, try it with an emotion
that you tend to struggle with, but not the most intense,
troublesome emotion. Remember that you are still learning, so begin with an easier task and work your way up to
the most difficult. If you aren't currently experiencing a
troublesome emotion, then you may need to bring one to
mind. In order to do this, think about a particular situation in which you feel the emotion or a particular difficulty
that you are currently having.

This exercise is suitable for women at all stages, whether
you are pregnant, a new mum or trying to conceive.

Mindfulness of emotion exercise

Get into a comfortable sitting position, ensuring that you have a straight back but allowing yourself to have a relaxed, comfortable posture. Settle into it. Gently close your eyes. Let your hands rest gently on your knees or in your lap.

Allow your mind to settle gently into the here and now.

Notice the sensations in your body ...

Feelings of touch or pressure where your body makes contact with the floor or the chair ...

Feelings of warmth or cool ...

The rhythm of your breathing ... the gentle in and out.

Notice the sensations as you breathe.

Use your breath as an anchor to connect to the here and now.

Bring to mind a particular unpleasant emotion. To do this you may need to think about a particular situation in which you feel that emotion, or a particular difficulty that you are having.

Recall the thoughts associated with that situation or difficulty and buy into them. Let them carry you away ...

Really immerse yourself in your thoughts and let the emotion take over.

Once the emotion is present, open yourself up to the sensations in your body.

Gently scan your body with your attention and find the areas in your body where the emotion feels the most intense or troublesome ...

Is it the feeling in your stomach?

Or maybe a tightness in your shoulders and neck?

Or perhaps a dull ache in your head?

Focus in on the most bothersome or intense sensation ...

Try to be curious and adventurous, as if you are interested in feeling everything that is involved in this sensation.

Explore the emotion by imagining that the sensations are an object ...

If the sensations were an object, what colour would it be?

What temperature would it be?

How would it feel to touch?

Would it be moving or stationary?

Would it be light or dense?

Approach the emotion with a sense of curiosity and acceptance.

Breathe gently around the emotion...

With every in-breath, find yourself growing bigger and making room for the emotion...

Notice that you are bigger than the emotion.

You might like to continue exploring the emotion by imagining that the emotion is an animal.

If the emotion were an animal, what would it look like?

How would it feel to touch?

Would it be moving or stationary?

Would it be light or heavy?

What would it be doing?

Try to develop a sense of kindness towards the emotion-animal...

Consider that even though it may be ugly or aggressive, it has got nowhere else to go.

Try to make room for the emotion...

This doesn't mean you have to like it or want it to be there...

It just means accepting it and allowing it to be there.

Spend some moments just sitting mindfully with the emotion...

Noticing the emotion...

Noticing your breathing.

When you are ready to end the exercise, do so gently, using your breathing as an anchor to bring your awareness with you back into the room...

In the exercise we tried two types of visual imagery: imagining the emotion as an object and imagining it as an animal. Sometimes people find one of these images more helpful than the other. Also, people often find that some emotions are best seen as objects and others as animals. You should use the imagery that works best for you. With time you may begin to use the same imagery for a particular emotion; always seeing anger as an angry, clawing cat for example. This can be helpful, as you can bring the image to mind quickly in your daily life.

My thoughts about *Mindfulness of emotions*:

....

....

....

....

....

....

EMOTIONS IN DAILY LIFE

You can use the waking up exercise, with a focus on emotion, to boost your acceptance of your emotions as you go about your daily life. Try the following exercise with your emotions throughout the day. It is suitable for women at all stages, whether you are pregnant, a new mum or trying to conceive.

Waking up exercise for emotion

First, notice your breathing.

Use your breathing as an anchor to the here and now.

Notice your emotions . . .

Notice where the emotion is sitting in your body . . .

Explore the emotion and, if it is helpful, visualise the emotion as an object or animal.

Gently open yourself up, making room for the emotion . . .

Accepting your emotional experiences moment by moment in your daily life is about going with the flow of your emotions. With greater awareness of your emotions moment by moment, you may notice that emotions tend to come and go naturally. At times our emotions may even fluctuate without any clear trigger, or in response to tiny details of our day. Understanding this may liberate you from feeling a need to read deep meaning into your moment-by-moment emotional experiences. For example, at the end of a day with a grizzly baby it is natural to experience feeling down, and having this experience may not be any reflection at all on you as a mum, nor on your baby.

It is important to be aware that the concept of being accepting of our emotions can be misinterpreted, and that there are some things that being accepting of our emotions does *not* mean. Being accepting of our emotions does not mean that we need to feel good about feeling anger, sadness or fear. It just means that we make room for these feelings when they arise. And if we also feel bad about the feelings, then we make room for that too.

It also does *not* mean that we shouldn't demonstrate self-care or have a breather when a situation is becoming heated. In future chapters, we will explore how to be kind to yourself and how to take care of yourself in depth. For now, just know that if you are having a bad day and feeling stressed, angry, sad or anxious then you deserve as much kindness and caring actions from yourself as you would give to your best friend.

Being aware and accepting of your emotions is completely consistent with also taking care of yourself. It is also consistent with having a break if a situation is becoming heated. No one is able to be 100 per cent accepting of and open to their emotions all the time. Even if you are a champion at acceptance, as a mum you are going to need to demonstrate these skills under extreme conditions! If you feel that an emotion is becoming intense and is threatening to take over, it is completely appropriate to take a break. For example, if a new mum who is struggling to settle her baby feels a rush of intense anger, it is entirely appropriate for her to put her baby in a safe place such as the baby's cot, or to give the baby to dad for a while, and have a breather. Even if the mother is confident that she won't lose control, it is still okay to take some time out in the name of self-care when experiencing a rush of an intense emotion. The mum may choose to practise mindfulness of emotions in a separate room away from the baby until she finds herself back in control, or she may engage in a self-care activity such as having a cup of tea, calling a friend to debrief or getting a breath of fresh air in her garden. If the mum does wish to continue settling her baby, then she may ensure that she is doing so in a manner that is most likely to take care of herself at the same time, such as by putting on some of her favourite music, taking her baby outside or rocking the baby in a rocking chair. By increasing your ability to be aware and accepting of your emotions, you increase your ability to catch these emotional waves early while you are still in control.

MY EMOTIONS, BABY'S EMOTIONS

Increasing your acceptance of your own emotions also benefits your baby in that it helps you to be aware and accepting of your baby as he is in the present moment. It enables you to become increasingly aware and accepting not just of your own emotions, but also of your baby's emotions. This acceptance provides an ideal environment for the baby's emotional development.

There are real connections between your baby's emotions and your own emotions. If your baby feels distressed, then this is likely to trigger distress in you. For many women, the sound of a baby crying, particularly their own baby crying, is the most gut-wrenching, heart-tearing sound imaginable. Of course, this is nature's way of telling us to identify what our baby needs, to provide it and to settle our child. This task is made more difficult, however, if we aren't accepting of our own emotions. Figuring out what a baby needs and settling the baby is not always easy. Your baby may seem to send mixed signals or no signals at all. It often involves a trial and error process ('Okay, your nappy is dry, so that isn't the problem. Is it a feed? Hmm, you fed only an hour ago so probably not. Are you tired? Maybe, let's try to put you to sleep then and we'll see how that goes . . .'). Some of the potential solutions can require persistence in the face of protest; for example, it can take persistent efforts with settling techniques to get a tired baby to sleep, and baby may protest strongly. Sometimes your baby may just seem to need a good cuddle, while at other times he may scream the house down no matter what you do. These are likely to be some of your most challenging times as a new mum.

If you have low awareness and acceptance of your own distress then you are likely to enter into a desperate and frantic race to make baby's distress go away as fast as possible ('Hurry, oh gosh I'll do anything, just make it stop!'). This frantic desperation works against the trial and error process. A mum can find herself quickly flitting from potential solution to potential solution without persisting long enough with anything that she is trying for it to really take effect. In the meantime, she is becoming increasing frantic. As she isn't accepting her distress as it is, her emotions may be multiplying and she may find herself also feeling anger, guilt or sadness. She may also be becoming increasingly desperate in her ideas about what may be causing her baby's distress. As a result she may be trying strategies that are less and less likely to work, when in reality a newborn baby's need is most likely to be either a feed, attention or affection, a change in stimulation or to be settled to sleep. (A nappy change or change of clothes for temperature are also possibilities, but because these are so easily ruled out, they don't tend to cause this kind of frantic desperation in mothers.)

The increasingly frantic distress of his mother is, of course, the last thing that baby needs to settle. If the mum can, instead, make room for her own distress as well as baby's distress, then an accepting, peaceful space is created for baby. This is much more likely to enable the baby to settle.

Why do babies rely upon us to settle them, anyway? When a baby experiences an emotion, he cannot be aware of, accepting of or understand that emotion. Babies cannot figure out what they need, let alone obtain what they need on their own, nor can they engage in self-care in order to soothe themselves. They simply don't have the skills. So what do babies do with emotions? In a sense, babies process their emotions by getting their mothers (or another caring adult) to process their emotions for them. Babies need the assistance of a caring adult to accept their emotional state, to soothe them when they are distressed and to meet the needs behind their emotions.

When seen this way, the long unsettled crying periods that most mums face make sense. Your baby doesn't just need a bit of emotional support and an occasional vent in the same way as your best friend or your partner. Rather, your baby needs you to process his emotions for him by accepting his emotions, making sense of his emotional state and meeting the needs that lie behind his distress.

ONE WOMAN'S STORY

Reading Rachel's story may help you to understand how acceptance of emotions can be a strength for a mum.

Rachel was already finding it difficult to cope with the emotional roller coaster of being the mother of a determined and active toddler, her son Nathan. So when she realised that she was pregnant with her second child she knew things had to change. Rachel had always been a sensitive and emotional person. At times she felt this had a positive side, making her kind and compassionate—surely a strength in a mum. At other times, though, she would become overwhelmed by her feelings. In these moments she would let her feelings take over and would find herself lashing out verbally, often at Nathan. Rachel knew how she wanted to handle challenges with Nathan and she had the skills to do it. But if she was overwhelmed by her feelings she would find herself, out of anger or frustration, doing exactly what she didn't want to do. She also realised that Nathan struggled with his own emotions (often resulting in temper tantrums) and wondered how she could support Nathan and her future baby in their own emotional development. Rachel felt that developing mindfulness of her emotions was the perfect solution.

Rachel practised mindfulness of emotions regularly throughout her pregnancy by visualising her emotions as an animal. She would focus her attention on the feeling of the emotion within her body and breathe into it, expanding her body to make room for the emotion. She found that she could sit with even painful emotions and make room for them. Rachel noticed that the more she practised mindfulness of emotions the more she was able to make room for her emotions in her everyday life. She began to find herself maintaining control of her actions in situations where she used to be overwhelmed by her feelings and act rashly.

It wasn't that her feelings were any less intense; rather, she made room for them, acknowledged them and hence she could do what she wanted to do. For example, one night Nathan absolutely refused to eat the dinner that she had prepared even though she had made a special effort to make one of his favourite meals. Rachel was furious and normally she'd have yelled at Nathan but her increased acceptance of her emotions gave her the space to act based on her values instead. Rachel didn't want to lose a nice evening as a family to raging at Nathan about eating his dinner, so she instead let her anger come and go, put Nathan's dinner into the freezer for another night and made him a toasted cheese sandwich instead. Rachel also noticed that her emotions were always changing. Feelings of sadness, anxiety, happiness and anger would come and go, sometimes without any clear trigger. Rachel realised that her feelings weren't a stable base on which to build her life.

When baby Lucy arrived, Rachel was relieved that she had put so much time into practising becoming more accepting of her emotions. In those first few days at home with baby Lucy Rachel experienced a tidal wave of baby blues as well as feelings of guilt, anger and frustration in her relationship with Nathan as she adjusted to being the mother of two. In the early days, Rachel often found herself weeping uncontrollably on the shoulder of her husband Matthew in the evenings. In the past she would have tried to fight the baby blues and the feelings of guilt and anger, struggling to be nothing but happy at this special time. Now, however, Rachel understood that her emotions were normal; the best thing to do was to allow herself to feel what she was feeling. Within the next three days the baby blues feelings came and went without any real triggers, until they finally went for good. As time went by she also adjusted to being the mother of two.

Rachel was also grateful for her skills at mindfulness of emotions when baby Lucy hit six weeks and began to have a regular 'witching hour' every evening at about 6 pm. Lucy would suddenly transform from a content, gorgeous little baby into a screaming, crying mess. Seeing baby Lucy in such distress tore Rachel's heart to pieces. She found herself needing to make room not just for her own distress but also for her baby's. Rachel would pause for a moment and imagine her distress as an animal, usually a tiger pacing in her ribcage, tearing at her heart. Then she would gently breathe and make room for it. This was made easier by considering that really, this was baby Lucy's tiger. It may be a vicious tiger and it may be tearing at her heart, but it belonged to her baby girl and it had nowhere else to go.

Rachel would start to feel sorry for the tiger, and this allowed her to make room for her feelings. She found that by accepting her feelings she was able to be patient and methodical in finding the best ways to soothe baby Lucy. After several nights she discovered that the best way of soothing her baby was to rock her in the rocking chair with relaxation music playing in the background. Every evening at 6pm Matthew would give Nathan a bath and prepare him for bed while Rachel rocked a distressed baby Lucy. It always took time and Rachel needed to be persistent, but eventually baby Lucy would calm. Rachel was confident that this was what Lucy needed—some quiet time, being soothed by her mum. She knew that her own heart was big enough to process Lucy's emotions too.

MY UNIQUE ADVENTURE
These comments may help you to understand how the information in this chapter might relate to your own unique experiences.

Help! This wasn't what I had planned!

May be relevant to women experiencing difficulty conceiving, miscarriage, complications, preterm birth, an unwanted birth experience or finding motherhood different from expectations.
There is so much about the journey to motherhood that we cannot precisely control. We cannot control aspects of how long it takes us to conceive; whether we have a miscarriage, complications or a preterm birth; how our birth unfolds; or exactly who our baby will be (gender, health or temperament). Yet we tend to plan these things out anyway! And when they don't go according to plan, we can experience an intense emotional reaction. We instinctively fight against reality or against our own emotions, but we cannot win these fights. Acceptance is about living in the situation as it actually is, in the here and now, and accepting our own emotional reaction to it. This doesn't mean that you have to like the situation or stop feeling disappointed, angry or sad. It just means accepting what is and accepting how we feel about it. When we accept how things are and how we feel, then we become empowered and can find the best way forward in accordance with our values.

How do I survive this?

May be relevant to women experiencing emotional challenges, tough physical symptoms such as morning sickness, or birth.
With regular practice of mindfulness of emotions we can become better at accepting our emotions and being more open to our emotional experiences as they are. This then can give us the resilience to face our challenges. We may understand that emotions, however painful, cannot harm or damage us. Instead of acting to dull our emotions, or blindly letting our emotions take over, we become free to act based on our values even in the most challenging times. During emotional times, such as when we experience the baby blues, we can go with the flow of our feelings, letting our emotions come and go without trying to read deep meanings into our temporary experience. Acceptance of emotions can also be a strength in times

of physical challenge, as our emotional reactions to physical symptoms often create an additional layer of distress.

If you would like to improve your ability to accept your emotions, commit to practising mindfulness of emotions. Even practising for five minutes a day may make a difference. Are you able to make room for your emotions? Are you able to let your feelings come and go? When you make room for your emotions, does it help you become the mum you want to be?

Grief and loss

May be relevant to any woman experiencing a loss, whether it be an obvious loss such as miscarriage or stillbirth, or the loss of pre-motherhood life, difficulty conceiving, an unwanted birth experience or motherhood being different from expectations.

Grief involves a painful mix of emotions, including sadness, anger and fear. Grief is also a natural and healthy process. Remember that pain and joy are attached. You need to open yourself up to feelings of grief associated with motherhood in order to also open yourself up to the joy and love associated with this journey. The choice is whether to close your heart to love and grief or to open it to these emotions. If you would like to open your heart to feelings of grief in order to open your heart to love, then practising mindfulness of emotions may be useful. You may find it allows you to express your feelings of grief, whether by connecting with others who have had similar experiences; talking about your feelings with your partner, family or friends; writing a letter, a story or a poem; or doing something concrete like planting a tree. Every person grieves in a unique way, so it is important to follow your own instincts in grieving.

Living with worry and anxiety

May be relevant to women with a history of anxiety, women struggling with anxiety or worries, or women with a specific worry about motherhood.

In order to take actions that matter to you, you may need to be willing to experience anxiety. But how do you become willing to experience anxiety? Practising mindfulness of emotions regularly can assist you in becoming more accepting of feelings of anxiety. Commit to practising this form of mindfulness regularly with your feelings of anxiety, even if just for five minutes a day. After several weeks of practising, see if you have noticed a difference in your willingness to experience anxiety. You can use the mindfulness of emotions exercise when you need to find willingness to experience anxiety in your everyday life. You may come to see your anxiety as a particular object or animal. Can you make room for anxiety if that is what it takes to become the mum that you want to be?

PUTTING IT INTO PRACTICE

✩ Notice how you tend to respond to your own emotions. Do your emotions tend to take over, causing you to do and say things that you didn't want to do or say? Do you find yourself struggling with your emotions and trying to get rid of them? What is the cost of this struggle?

✩ If you think that you would benefit from being more accepting of your own emotions, then commit to practising mindfulness of emotions regularly, even if for just five minutes a day. Are you able to make room for unpleasant emotions? Remember that you are making room for your unpleasant emotions in order to be the mum that you want to be.

✩ Practise making room for your unpleasant emotions in your daily life. When an unpleasant emotion arises, take a breath and, while you breathe, feel yourself getting bigger and making room for the emotion. If it helps, you can imagine that the emotion is an object or an animal.

✩ Notice your emotional experiences in your daily life. Do your emotions tend to come and go?

8

When the here and now is physically painful

Becoming a mum involves moments of, let's be honest, sheer agony. Obviously, there's the pain of childbirth. But there are other forms of physical pain and discomfort too, such as morning sickness, reflux and backache during pregnancy, healing of tears and scars in the postpartum period and cracked or damaged nipples if you are breastfeeding. These times of physical pain and discomfort also often occur with emotional highs and lows.

So how can you best manage the physical pain? In this chapter, we explore how to live through the moments of physical pain and discomfort. In doing so, we draw upon the skills we have learned in the previous chapters, such as mindfulness, as well as upon your values as a mum.

MINDFULNESS AND PHYSICAL PAIN OR DISCOMFORT

At first glance, it may seem like mindfulness is exactly what you don't need when the here and now involves physical pain or discomfort. However, a mindfulness approach to physical pain or discomfort can in fact be beneficial. Moments of intense physical pain are often worsened by focusing on anxious thoughts about the pain, imagining it persisting in the future, and then becoming entangled in thoughts about our own ability to cope with it. Dwelling on thoughts about our physical pain often also increases our emotional distress. Moreover, both our anxious thoughts and our emotional distress can actually heighten our sensations of pain, as they can change the way our brain responds to the pain signals. A mindfulness approach to physical pain or discomfort can therefore be helpful, because we can stop ourselves from becoming caught in a spiral of catastrophic thoughts and our own emotional reactions to them, and instead bring ourselves back to living through the pain just one moment at a time. In this state, our brain is more likely respond to pain signals in a way that dampens our continued sensations of pain; for example, by releasing natural endorphins.

Instead of focusing on our discomfort, we can use mindfulness to turn our attention to something simple, like our breathing. For example, a birthing woman may use mindfulness to keep her attention on her breathing during each contraction. As she feels the contractions getting more painful, thoughts may arise such as 'I can't cope' or 'how long will this last?' Using mindfulness, the woman can notice these thoughts for what they are, just thoughts, and bring her attention back to her breathing. In this way, she can give birth one contraction at a time.

A mindfulness approach can also be used to focus our attention on a positive activity even though we are experiencing discomfort. For example, a woman might be reading a favourite novel while she experiences morning sickness. Mindfulness may help her to bring her attention back to the novel and to enjoy reading rather than dwelling on her thoughts and feelings about her nausea. A mindfulness approach to physical pain can also be helpful, because we instinctively tend to brace against physical pain and this bracing can tense up muscles, causing more pain. Mindfulness can be used to deliberately soften into our pain, ensuring that we don't magnify the pain by bracing against it.

It is important to note that taking a mindful approach to physical pain/discomfort does not mean that you have to, or should, live through pain when there are steps that you can take to obtain relief from it. Having the skill to soften into and accept physical pain/discomfort does not mean that it is better or more virtuous to experience pain than to take steps to avoid it. What it does mean is that we should take whatever steps we feel comfortable with taking, in line with our values, in order to obtain relief from the pain, and then use our mindfulness skills to soften into the pain or discomfort that is left without being caught up in dire thoughts about it. In other words, the approach is simply to do whatever you can that is consistent with your values, and be mindful of the rest. Thus, you should investigate fully your options for pain relief, both pharmacological and non-pharmacological (including positions, heat packs and showers), for labour and also for any other pains that you experience during pregnancy, birth and the postpartum period. These options should be discussed with your midwife or doctor. You can then make informed choices about what pain relief is best for you based on your values and in your circumstances. Also remember that you may need to be flexible, depending on exactly how your pregnancy, birth and postpartum experience unfold.

The following mindfulness of breathing exercise is adapted for use during moments of physical pain or discomfort. Practising mindfulness of breathing regularly will enhance your ability to be mindful in the painful moments.

Mindfulness of breathing exercise for pain

Allow your mind to settle into the here and now.

Settle, gently, into noticing your breathing.

Notice the rhythm of your breathing ... the gentle in and out ...

Notice every breath ... in and out.

If your mind wanders or if thoughts arise, notice these thoughts and gently bring your attention back to your breathing.

With every in-breath feel yourself getting bigger, making room for the painful sensations.

Feel each breath softening around the pain ...

Allow your body to gently settle, as if relaxing into the pain.

You may find it helpful to visualise the pain as an object or an animal.

Notice the pain's colour, texture, temperature, behaviour.

Make room for the pain as best you can, perhaps by contemplating how this pain is part of your body nurturing your baby and bringing your baby into the world.

Focus on your breathing ...

All you have to do is breathe ...

In and out ...

When you are ready to end the exercise, do so gently, bringing awareness with you back into the room ...

This mindfulness exercise can be practised regularly in the lead-up to experiences such as giving birth.

My thoughts on *Mindfulness of breathing for pain*:

....

....

....

....

....

....

LIVING THROUGH IT

Moments of physical pain and discomfort can feel overwhelming. We may find ourselves weeping uncontrollably, wishing we could change reality, or thinking thoughts like 'I can't do this'. In fact, moments of physical pain and discomfort are a natural part of the unfolding experience of motherhood. In a sense, there is nothing to be coped with and nothing to be done. Most of the moments of physical pain or discomfort that a woman experiences in becoming a mum are her body doing what it needs to do in order to bring her baby into the world. In that sense, the pain is normal and healthy. These moments of normal, healthy physical pain and discomfort will pass naturally with time. All you need to do is to live through them.

Your mind may jump in with the thought, 'I can't possibly live through this pain!' But think about this honestly for a moment. Isn't it the case that all you need to do in order to survive the bouts of healthy pain that are a normal part of becoming a mum, is just to let time pass? Again, this does not in any way mean that you can't or shouldn't access available pain relief. It also doesn't mean that you won't find yourself crying, shouting or screaming. In reality, crying, shouting, screaming—even saying 'I can't cope'—are all normal and healthy ways to cope during intensely painful moments. If you don't believe me, have a chat to your midwife or doctor and ask them how many times they have heard a labouring woman shout, 'I can't do this!'—and then watched her do it.

There are many ways to cope with pain, so it is helpful if we can hold lightly our thoughts about how well we are coping. Instead, focus on simply living through the experience. How do you live through a painful experience? By taking it a moment at a time. Take a breath. Then take another. Just keep breathing.

DRAW STRENGTH FROM YOUR VALUES

It is easier to experience physical pain/discomfort if you are doing so for a reason. You can draw the strength to live through experiences of pain/discomfort by thinking of them as part of becoming the mum that you want to be. There is far greater dignity in bravely and willingly facing moments of pain in the name of one's values than in being a victim, dragged through life by pain. By remembering your values as a mum and choosing to have the pain that you are experiencing, if this is another step towards becoming the mother that you want to be, you can find the strength to keep going.

You might like to remind yourself of your values as a mum by writing them down and putting them somewhere that you see every day, or simply by pausing and reminding yourself why you are taking this journey. For example, many women experience the pain of damaged nipples in the first month postpartum as they are establishing breastfeeding and their baby is learning how to feed properly. If you strongly value breastfeeding, then reminding yourself of your values in relation to breastfeeding (such as the health benefits to your baby, convenience in the long term or promoting bonding) may help you to persist through the pain.

You may like to develop some 'mummy mantras' to remind yourself of your values during painful moments. These mantras may be unique to you or to the situation. You may find it particularly useful to address the mantra towards your baby.

Some examples include:

☆ 'I take this nausea on willingly so that you may be healthy and well'

☆ 'I am facing this because I am a mother'

☆ 'I take on this pain so that you may live'

☆ 'I am willing to experience this pain if that's what it takes to breastfeed my baby'

☆ 'I face each contraction knowing it brings my baby closer'.

List some mummy mantras that you could find helpful:

....

....

....

....

....

....

....

....

BE KIND TO YOURSELF

During times of physical pain or discomfort, be kind to yourself. These aren't the times to be trying to achieve a list of goals; these are the times to indulge yourself. It can be beneficial to keep your focus on a positive activity, as this can assist you to avoid dwelling on your discomfort, and can help to boost your mood.

It is particularly important to be kind to yourself in times of physical pain or discomfort that require endurance, such as if you are enduring weeks of morning sickness. These periods may be perfect for indulging in some of your favourite activities, such as reading favourite novels, watching favourite shows or movies or listening to favourite music. Any activity that you truly love and that is likely to keep you engrossed and positive may be beneficial. Your mindfulness skills will help you to keep your attention on the positive activity.

Some ways that I can indulge during times of physical pain/discomfort are (remember to consider not only birth but also morning sickness, aches and pains during pregnancy, healing after birth and learning to breastfeed):

....

....

....

....

....

....

....

ONE WOMAN'S STORY

Reading Maya's story may help you to find ways to cope with physical pain and discomfort.

Maya had dreadful morning sickness. It began as a queasy feeling before she'd even taken the pregnancy test to confirm that she had fallen pregnant, and by seven weeks she was constantly nauseous. Maya was vomiting half a dozen times a day. She tried all the usual remedies such as ginger, peppermints and eating crackers before she got out of bed each morning, but she still felt dreadfully sick.

Sometimes, after vomiting up yet another meal, she would burst into tears. Maya found herself having thoughts like, 'I can't cope with this' and 'I won't survive'. She knew, though, that there was no such thing as coping or not coping. Whether she liked it or not, each day would go by, she would feel nauseous, she would vomit and eventually the morning sickness would settle.

Maya drew strength from her values. She had read that some scientists think that morning sickness evolved to protect unborn babies from substances in our adult diet that could be harmful to them. Maya liked the idea that her nausea and vomiting, though unpleasant, were her body's way of protecting her vulnerable baby by (rather forcefully!) ensuring that she didn't eat anything potentially dangerous for her baby and that she spent much of her time resting and sleeping. She decided that, as dreadful as the morning sickness was, she wanted to protect her baby and that she was willing to have the morning sickness if that was what it took. Sometimes, after vomiting or when the nausea was particularly bad, she'd remind herself of this by saying, 'I'm doing this for my baby'. Maya kept herself positive by indulging in reading her favourite books and watching her favourite television shows. With time, the pregnancy progressed and the morning sickness passed.

Maya also found herself needing to draw strength from her values when giving birth. Again, she reminded herself that she was going through the pain for her baby, saying to herself, 'I'm feeling this pain so that my baby will be born' and 'every contraction brings my baby closer'. Maya focused her attention on her breathing, especially during contractions. If she found herself having thoughts about how long the labour would last or how painful it would become, she would pull her attention back to her breathing in the here and now. She took the labour one contraction at a time. To Maya's way of thinking, she didn't need to give birth. Not all at once, anyway. She just needed to get through the next contraction. Maya also decided to use the gas to manage her pain during the birth, and she found this helpful too. She used what she could, while still remaining faithful to her values, in order to manage her pain.

Maya found that it took six weeks for baby Amelia to learn how to breastfeed well. While baby Amelia was still mastering how to latch on properly, she would munch on and damage Maya's nipples, making them very sore for the next feed. Maya found that, despite the pain, she was able to persist with breastfeeding because she kept reminding herself why she was doing it—that is, because of her own values regarding the health benefits that breastfeeding gave to Amelia and also the bonding time with her during feeds. This gave Maya the strength to live through the pain.

MY UNIQUE ADVENTURE
These comments may help you to understand how the information in this chapter might relate to your own unique experiences.

How do I survive this?
May be relevant to women experiencing emotional challenges, challenging physical symptoms such as morning sickness, or birth. What does it mean to cope with challenging physical symptoms like morning sickness or the physical pain of childbirth? Sometimes our minds chime in with thoughts like 'I can't survive this' or 'I can't cope', but we need to remember that living through such experiences is really just that: living through them. If you are experiencing physical symptoms or pain, then take whatever steps you can, in line with your values, to obtain relief from this. If you are unsure of your options for pain relief, discuss these with your midwife or doctor. Bring yourself back into contact with your values and allow yourself to draw strength from them. See if you can face the pain

willingly for your baby. Then take a breath. Take another. Just keep on breathing and let yourself live through it.

PUTTING IT INTO PRACTICE

✧ It is almost certain that your journey to motherhood will involve moments of physical pain and discomfort. Plan ahead for these moments. For example, you may like to consider the options available to manage physical pain during birth that are consistent with your values, and discuss them with your midwife or doctor.

✧ How can you remind yourself of your values during the painful and challenging times? Take some time to find the right mummy mantras for you and try them. Does it help to remind yourself why you are experiencing the pain that you are experiencing?

✧ How might you use mindfulness during the painful times? You might like to practise mindfulness of breathing regularly so that you are already skilled at using it when you need it during times of physical pain. You may also find that mindfulness of thoughts or mindfulness of emotions exercises are useful.

✧ The moments of physical pain or discomfort are times to indulge yourself. How can you indulge yourself during these moments?

9

Loving
baby

You are probably aware that a mother's love, demonstrated in small ways moment by moment, day by day, sets a baby up for a lifetime of psychological health. Yet, what exactly do we mean by love? What is it exactly that a mum does when she loves her baby, and how can we ensure, as mums, that we do that? In this chapter we will explore the concept of love, concluding that the love your baby needs involves acceptance and kindness. Through specific exercises we aim to practise taking an accepting and kind stance towards ourselves and our baby, thus learning to give our baby the love that she needs, even in difficult circumstances.

WHAT IS A MOTHER'S LOVE?

In the English language we use the word 'love' in a number of different ways. So, what does a mother mean when she says that she loves her baby? One meaning of the word 'love' is that the loved person, thing or experience brings us feelings of happiness, joy and pleasure. This is what we mean when we say that we love an object or an experience. It is also one of the ways in which we love other people (though it isn't the only meaning of love when it comes to other people, as we will see in a moment). Mothers often have the experience of their baby, their loved one, bringing them feelings of pleasure and joy. This aspect of love, then, is built out of feelings.

Feelings, as you may well have noticed from practising mindfulness of your emotions, are transitory. All feelings come and go, and so we cannot expect a thing or a person that we love to bring us feelings of joy, happiness and pleasure all the time. For example, you may well have had the experience during the first trimester of pregnancy of some of your most loved foods suddenly bringing you no joy at all. Similarly, we also cannot expect our baby to bring us constant feelings of happiness, joy or pleasure. Sometimes we can become trapped in the idea that we should constantly feel happiness, joy and pleasure around our baby and that our baby should never trigger feelings of sadness, anger or fear. This is simply unrealistic. Just as you wouldn't want to eat chocolate constantly, there may be times when you would like a break from your baby. This doesn't mean that you don't love your baby.

You can encourage this aspect of love for your baby by giving yourself the space for the feelings of happiness, joy and pleasure to grow. Do this by staying psychologically present with your baby in daily life—that is, by being mindful. The pleasures and the joy associated with your baby exist in the present moment, the here and now. When you take the time to notice your baby as she is in the here and now, you are more likely to notice the little things about your baby that you enjoy; and gradually, over time, these moments of joy knit themselves into loving feelings. It makes sense to cultivate this aspect of love for your baby because if your baby brings you joy, this will make being a mum more rewarding for you.

However, this aspect of love is only a small part of what we mean when we talk about loving other people, and it is these other aspects of love that your baby needs. When we talk about loving another human being we also mean that we value and accept that human being as they are, and that we wish for their happiness even if that doesn't bring us happiness, joy or pleasure ourselves. Many mothers find that they care more about the happiness of their baby than their own happiness. This is the meaning of love when we say, 'Love makes the world go round' or 'All you need is love' or 'Love your neighbour', and this is the love that your baby needs from you. This love includes a sense of acceptance—of accepting the person as they are. It also includes kindness, as it involves wishing that person well. This aspect of love is not built of feelings; rather, it is a stance that you may take towards a person. It is possible to love someone in this sense and at the very same time feel strong, negative feelings such as anger towards that person.

Unlike feelings, which are transitory, taking a loving stance towards a person can be done completely and unconditionally. It is this kind of love that benefits your baby. This kind of love creates a safe, nurturing space in which baby can grow, and teaches your baby to approach herself with acceptance and kindness.

BECOMING AN ACCEPTING SPACE FOR YOUR BABY

An important aspect of love is acceptance. This means accepting your baby as he is. This kind of acceptance isn't about how you feel about your baby; rather, it is a stance that you can choose to take towards your baby. During the times that your baby triggers emotions in you such as sadness, anger or fear, taking an accepting stance towards your baby is about allowing your baby to be who he is and allowing your emotions to be there too. It is about accepting your baby, and accepting that sometimes your baby triggers feelings of sadness, anger or fear and that this is okay too.

When you become this kind of accepting space for your baby, you provide your baby with a safe and secure environment to grow. You also encourage your baby to develop self-acceptance. Fortunately, you can improve your ability to be accepting with practice. The following exercises focus on taking an accepting stance towards your baby. The exercises build upon the mindfulness exercises we learned in the previous chapters. The first version of the exercise is suitable for women who are pregnant and the second is for new mums. If you are still trying to conceive, put these exercises to the side for now.

Accepting space exercise (for pregnancy)
Get into a comfortable position.
Let your mind settle gently into the here and now.
Use your breathing as an anchor to connect to the present moment.
Place your hands on your belly and bring your attention to your pregnant belly.
Notice the weight of your baby inside you . . .
Notice the feeling of carrying another, of carrying your child.
Notice what your baby is doing . . .
Is your baby moving? If so gently bring your attention to his movements, to his kicks and turns and rolls.
If your baby isn't moving, notice that he is quiet at the moment. Maybe he is sleeping.
As you breathe each in-breath, feel your breathing gently swirl around your baby and caress him.
Gently, as best you can, open yourself to your baby.
It is like flinging yourself wide open . . .
As if you are as boundless as the sky . . .
Notice that your heart is big enough to contain all of your baby's possibilities and potentials.
Notice that your heart is big enough to contain all the thoughts and feelings that your baby triggers in you, the pleasant and the unpleasant.
If unpleasant thoughts or feelings are present, gently open yourself to them. You don't have to like them or want them to be there, you just need to make room for them.
With every in-breath, feel your heart opening and widening for your baby.
See if you can be open to your baby exactly as he is . . .
This doesn't mean that you need to like everything about how your mothering journey is unfolding, it just means that you are making room in your heart for your baby.
When you are ready to end the exercise, do so gently, bringing your increased acceptance of your baby with you into your everyday life . . .

This exercise can help you to practise taking an accepting stance towards your baby. The next version of the exercise is for new mums. You can do this exercise while you are with your baby. It is best to try the exercise for the first time when your baby is in a calm state, because this is likely to be easier for you. However, it is fantastic to practise when your baby is unsettled too. After all, it is when your baby is unsettled that it is going to be the most challenging to accept your baby exactly as she is.

Accepting space exercise (for new mums)

Let your mind settle gently into the here and now.

Use your breathing as an anchor to connect to the present moment.

Bring your attention to focus on your baby.

Perhaps your baby is in your arms or maybe you are watching your baby in her cot or on a rug.

Slowly cast your eyes over your baby, noticing the details of her body, noticing her toes, her legs, her arms and hands, her little fingers, noticing her face and the details of her features ...

Really pay attention to your baby, as if you are seeing her again for the very first time.

If your baby is in your arms, notice the weight of your baby and the feeling of your baby against your skin.

If your baby is in her cot or on a rug, you might like to gently touch your baby, noticing how it feels to connect to your baby with touch.

You might like to smell your baby, noticing her unique baby smell.

Notice your baby's breathing, the gentle rhythm of your baby's in- and out-breaths.

Gently, as best you can, open yourself to your baby ...

It is like flinging yourself wide open ...

As if you are as boundless as the sky.

Notice that your heart is big enough to contain all of your baby; even your baby's fussiness, your baby's problem feeds, your baby's sleeping problems, the way your baby came into the world.

Notice that your heart is big enough to contain all the thoughts and feelings that your baby triggers in you, the pleasant and the unpleasant.

If unpleasant thoughts or feelings are present, gently open yourself to them. You don't have to like them or want them to be there, you just need to make room for them.

With every in-breath, feel your heart opening and widening for your baby. See if you can be open to your baby exactly as your baby is …

This doesn't mean that you need to like everything your baby does; it doesn't mean you have to like everything about how your mothering journey is unfolding; it just means that you are making room in your heart for your baby.

When you are ready to end the exercise, do so gently, bringing your increased acceptance of your baby with you into your everyday life …

With increased practice you can become better and better at being an accepting space for your baby. Notice that being an accepting space for your baby means that you also need to become an accepting space for yourself. This includes accepting your own thoughts and feelings. Becoming an accepting space for baby isn't about trying to force yourself to feel a particular way about your baby. Rather, it involves becoming an accepting space for your baby as she is and for yourself as you are (including your thoughts and feelings). You may need to use the skills learned in previous chapters relating to thoughts and feelings in order to do this.

My thoughts on becoming an accepting space:

. . . .

. . . .

. . . .

. . . .

. . . .

. . . .

. . . .

. . . .

KINDNESS FOR BABY

In addition to acceptance, a mother's love also involves kindness—which really means wishing for your baby's happiness. You may find that a sense of kindness towards your baby develops easily and naturally, or you may find that you can benefit from some practice. You may also find that a sense of kindness towards your baby usually comes easily, but that it can be challenging when your baby is unsettled at 3 am!

Most mothers find that they have a natural head start in developing kindness for their baby. It is often easier for a mum to be kind towards her own baby than kind towards anyone else. However, mums also find that their baby challenges their kindness more than anyone else does, and that they need to find kindness for their baby under extreme conditions. As a result, even the kindest mum may find that she benefits from learning to cultivate kindness consciously towards her baby.

The following exercise involves practising developing kindness for your baby, and is suitable for women trying to conceive, women who are pregnant or new mums. In the exercise you imagine that your baby is in front of you. If you are still trying to conceive, simply imagine your future baby. If you are pregnant you can imagine your baby as he is now in your womb, or you can imagine your baby as a newborn. As this exercise involves visual imagery, it is best done with your eyes closed.

Kindness for baby exercise

Get into a comfortable sitting position, ensuring that you have a straight back but allowing yourself to have a relaxed, comfortable posture. Settle into it. Gently close your eyes. Let your hands rest gently on your knees or in your lap.

Allow your mind to settle gently into the here and now.

Notice the sensations in your body ...

Feelings of touch or pressure where your body makes contact with the floor or the chair ...

Feelings of warmth or cool …
The rhythm of your breathing …
The gentle in and out.
Notice the sensations as you breathe.
Use your breath as an anchor to connect to the here and now.
Start to visualise a ball of warm light in your heart …
This warm light is kindness, compassion, openness.
Imagine your baby, as he is now or as a newborn …
Imagine your baby as he is, with all of the history that you and your baby share, and with all of the potentials and possibilities that your baby has.
Allow yourself to acknowledge the positive aspects and the negative aspects of your history with your baby, as well as the positive and the negative future possibilities.
With all of that present, try, as best you can, to allow yourself to feel kindness towards your baby, to wish for your baby's happiness.
Allow the ball of warm light to grow and radiate out, bathing your baby in kindness.
Imagine that this warm glowing light is exactly what your baby needs, and it is filling your baby.
Continue to radiate warmth and light towards your baby …
If you are feeling stuck, you may like to imagine that you are someone who symbolises kindness to you.
You can imagine that you are a spiritual figure, or a fictional character, or someone you know.
As best you can, continue to radiate warmth and light towards your baby …
As your baby fills with more and more light, your baby's heart also develops a warm, glowing ball of light.
This glowing ball of light reflects back to you, and you feel yourself filling up with the warm, glowing light from your baby …
When you are ready to end the exercise, do so gently, using your breathing as a anchor to bring your awareness with you back into the room. Try to bring this sense of kindness for you baby with you …

With practice you will find it easier to cultivate a sense of kindness towards your baby. You can use the visualisation in your daily life to give yourself a boost of kindness towards your baby when you are finding the need to show kindness under extreme conditions.

My thoughts on the *Kindness for baby* exercise:

....

....

....

....

....

....

LOVE IN ACTION

How is this love expressed day by day? If you take an accepting and kind stance towards your baby but don't express this in action, it doesn't really benefit your baby. Love in action is about transforming this loving stance into responding, as best you can, to your baby's needs. This starts with an awareness of your baby that allows you to notice your baby's cues. With openness to your baby as she is, you can begin to notice your baby's cues and behaviours. Based on her cues, you may form ideas about what your baby is feeling (sleepy, hungry, unsettled) and what she might need. From a sense of kindness, you may try giving your baby what you think she needs (being settled to sleep, a feed or a cuddle). As you do so, continue to be aware of and open to your baby. Does this seem to be what she needed? Notice that this is a trial and error process, but its bedrock is an open, aware and kind stance towards your baby.

If you are a new mum, how can you show love to your baby day by day? What needs do you notice? What cues does your baby show? How can you respond? If you are still trying to conceive or are pregnant, how do you think you can show love to your baby when she is born?

....

....

....

....

....

A DEVELOPING BOND

You may be aware that chickens will bond with ('imprint') any moving object that is available in the first few days after hatching. A chicken will then, forever after, recognise this object as its mother. As a result, it is absolutely vital for a chicken to be with its mother after hatching if they are to develop a normal bond.

In contrast, the bond between a human mother and a baby develops over time. Sometimes we can get so caught up in how nice it is (when possible) to enjoy the moments after birth by cuddling and feeding our newborn baby that we can start to think that these moments are vital to our ability to bond with our baby. We can also start to think that we must fall in love with our baby in these moments after birth, or we'll have missed the opportunity to bond forever. Fortunately, however, this is not the case. We, unlike chickens, do not have a limited window of opportunity to bond with our babies. We have infinite chances.

The bond between a mum and her baby is just as complex, rich and beautiful as any other bond between two humans. The bond between a mother and her baby can and does develop in a hundred different ways. Just as there are couples who claim to have fallen in love at first sight, and best friends who say that they connected straight away, so there are mums who had a similar experience of falling in love with their baby in a rush. On the other hand, just as there are couples who fell in love gradually over months or even years, and best friends who connected gradually after much time spent together, so there are mums who had a similar experience falling in love with their baby gradually over time. It is not better or worse to fall in love with your baby quickly or gradually. Even if you fall in love quickly, your baby's birth may not be the moment that it happens. There are many women who fell in love with their baby at other moments, such as when they found out that they were pregnant, when they first saw their baby at a scan, when they first felt their baby move, when their baby first smiled or when their baby first babbled to them. The diversity and complexity of human love is a positive thing because you actually have infinite chances to develop and strengthen the love between yourself and your baby. No matter where you are on the journey to motherhood, if you can open yourself up to your baby as he is then you can begin to notice all of the unique, individual characteristics of your baby. Over time, these observations will knit themselves into loving feelings. It doesn't matter exactly when this happens.

Of course, the other side of the bond is your baby and your baby's need for a loving mum. From your baby's perspective, your bond is built over time from many repetitions of mum lovingly responding to baby's needs. For your baby this is what matters—that you notice your baby's needs and that you, as best you can, respond to them. Your baby really doesn't care how you feel about him at any given moment, just that you lovingly respond. It is the loving stance, the stance of acceptance and kindness that your baby needs from you.

ONE WOMAN'S STORY

Reading Maria's story may help you to fall in love with your own baby and to give your baby the love (acceptance and kindness) that your baby needs.

Maria didn't connect with her baby Marco straight away. After a long and painful labour, Maria was utterly exhausted. Looking at her newborn baby Marco lying on her chest, covered in vernix and blood from the birth and with a strange cone-shaped head from being pushed through the birth canal, Maria didn't find herself overcome with feelings of love. Baby Marco looked more like an alien than the beautiful baby that she had been imagining. Besides, all she had the strength to feel was relief that the birth was over.

When Maria and baby Marco came home from hospital days later, Maria still didn't feel a rush of love while looking at her baby. For the time being she still felt exhausted, sore and overwhelmed by the baby blues. At first she felt guilty that her motherly love hadn't kicked in yet. But her husband Francesco reassured her. He pointed out that, in spite of how perfect they were for each other, it had taken him months of persistent wooing to get Maria to see it. Francesco figured that Maria was just someone who took her time to fall in love and that she should relax, enjoy motherhood, and give Marco time to woo her too. Maria decided that she would do just that.

Although loving feelings hadn't kicked in yet, Maria was able to love baby Marco by opening herself up to him and by responding kindly to his needs. She deliberately spent time each day just noticing Marco. She would watch him sleeping, noticing his expressions, smelling his unique baby smell and feeling his touch. Maria opened herself up to baby Marco as he was. She knew that she could, as his mum, accept him as he was in the here and now, no matter how she felt about him at any given moment.

Maria also practised cultivating kindness towards her baby. She visualised the kindness as a ball of warm light radiating from her heart towards Marco. She would imagine that the warm light filled baby Marco and that it was exactly what he needed. During the day she kept herself open to baby Marco as he was, noticing his cues for feeds and for sleeps. She also responded with kindness to baby Marco's needs, offering him a feed when he was hungry, giving him a cuddle when he needed to be settled and rocking him off to sleep when he was tired. She knew that she was meeting Marco's need for a loving mum.

Gradually, over time, Maria felt more and more moments of warm feelings towards baby Marco. She would find herself thinking about how delicious he smelt, or enjoying the feeling of cuddling him, or thinking that he looked particularly cute in a new outfit. Marco gradually became more and more like a little human being. He started to smile and make cooing noises. Maria also began to see more resemblances between Francesco and Marco. She noticed that her baby had the same shaped face, the same chocolate brown eyes and the same cheeky grin as his father. Then, when baby Marco was 12 weeks old, he laughed. He laughed a big, generous belly laugh. Maria's heart melted, and she knew that she loved him.

MY UNIQUE ADVENTURE
These comments may help you to understand how the information in this chapter might relate to your own unique experiences.

Adoption
May be relevant to mums waiting to adopt or new mums of adopted babies.
The development of love between a mother and her baby is just as complicated, unique and beautiful a process as the development of love between any two human beings. There are a million ways to fall in love with your baby. If you are still waiting to adopt, allow yourself to indulge in imagining your baby, in all of his or her awesome possibilities. There will be a unique, precious baby just for you. If you are a new mum, then open your heart to your baby in the here and now. Allow yourself and your baby time for your relationship to develop and your love to unfold. Let yourself enjoy falling in love.

Becoming Mum ... again
May be relevant to women with older children who are pregnant or have a new baby.
No matter what your relationship with your older children has been like so far, you have the opportunity to nurture a strong,

loving bond with them, starting today. Try practising the accepting space and kindness exercises in this chapter, focusing on your older children. Can you find room in your heart for your children as they are, including their faults, mistakes and tantrums? Can you find kindness for your children? Remember that from your children's point of view, a loving bond is created through many repetitions of you lovingly responding to their needs. How do you respond to the needs of your children? How do you show your love for them?

You also need to remember to give your older children time to fall in love with their new sibling. Accepting any negative feelings that they may have about the new baby, or the changes in their life, as normal and natural will help your children to keep their hearts open to the changes, including learning to love their sibling.

Help! This wasn't what I had planned!
May be relevant to women experiencing difficulty conceiving, miscarriage, pregnancy complications, preterm birth, an unwanted birth experience or finding motherhood different from expectations.

When you find unexpected challenges or difficulties on the journey to motherhood, or when it unfolds in a way that you didn't expect, this can sometimes disrupt, for a time, the development of loving feelings towards your baby. First, remember that this disruption is not permanent and it is not your fault. The development of love between a mum and her baby is just as complicated, unique and beautiful a process as the development of love between any two human beings. There are many ways to fall in love with your baby. It is important, as soon as you can, to practise staying psychologically present with your baby.

Also remember that there are a million little opportunities to fall in love with your baby, and they all exist in the here and now. It can be tempting to avoid any unpleasant feelings that you may have about your baby or about your transition to being a mum. It may even seem like you have to get rid of the pain in order to develop loving feelings towards your baby. However, all you actually need to do is open your heart; this will allow both the pain and your baby in.

Finally, it is also important to remember that the love your baby needs from you is acceptance and kindness. It is possible to be accepting and kind towards your baby while you are waiting to fall in love with him. You may find it helpful to regularly practise cultivating acceptance and kindness towards your baby.

Grief and loss

May be relevant to any woman experiencing a loss, whether it be an obvious loss such as miscarriage or stillbirth, or the loss of pre-motherhood life, difficulty conceiving, an unwanted birth experience, or motherhood being different from expectations.

When you have experienced a loss in the past or the present, it can be tempting to try to block out the pain of your grief. Perhaps you may find yourself unwilling to form an attachment to your baby because this makes you vulnerable to the pain of losing her. This takes us back to what we learnt in Chapter 2. In life, pain and joy are attached. In order to have the joy of love, you need to open your heart to the pain of loss as well. Are you able to open your heart to your baby as she is, including the vulnerabilities, including the fact that you may lose her? If you have lost your baby, are you able to give your lost baby space in your heart even though it is painful? If you would like to try you may find it helpful to practise the accepting space exercise given in this chapter.

Young mums and unplanned pregnancies

May be relevant to young mothers, younger-than-planned mothers and women experiencing an unplanned pregnancy.

If you are experiencing an unplanned pregnancy, you may find that you fall in love with your baby later in your journey to motherhood. It is important to remember that this is normal. As best you can, open your heart to your baby as he is in the here and now, as well as to any doubts, fears, or regrets that you may have about your pregnancy. It may be tempting to try to push away your doubts, fears or regrets. It may seem like you have to do this in order to learn to love your baby. This is about remembering what we discovered in Chapter 2—that the pain and the joy are attached. In fact, you need to open your heart to any doubts, fears or regrets in order to also open your heart to your baby. You may find it helpful to practise the accepting space exercise given in this chapter. There are infinite opportunities to fall in love with your baby.

PUTTING IT INTO PRACTICE

✩ If you are currently pregnant or are a new mum, notice times when you are an open, accepting space for your baby and times when you close yourself off to your baby as she is in the here and now. What are the differences between these times? If you notice yourself closing yourself off to your baby, gently open yourself up again. Can you choose to accept your baby as she is?

✩ Practise cultivating kindness towards your baby by imagining your kindness as a ball of warm light radiating towards your baby. You can do this if you are still trying to conceive by simply imaging your future baby. Even if you find that you usually feel kindness towards your baby and that it comes easily, remember that your baby will challenge you! The more you practise finding kindness for your baby the easier it will be to find it in the middle of the night.

✩ If you are a new mum, observe little ways to put your love into action by noticing your baby's needs and responding to them.

✩ If you are still trying to conceive or are pregnant, find a way to show your love for your baby now. Can you show your love for your baby by talking or singing to her? By protecting her? By preparing for her arrival?

10

Taking care
of yourself

How would you react if you found someone in your baby's nursery knowingly destroying your baby's belongings? Surely you would be angry and leap to your baby's defence. How would you react if you received a letter from the government saying that your baby would not receive an education? Surely you'd be outraged at the opportunities that would be denied to your baby. You would be conscious of the impact of an education on his future wellbeing and happiness and you'd quickly leap to defend his future prospects.

As a mum, one of your roles is to defend your baby's rights. This includes defending your baby's future wellbeing and happiness, and this means strongly defending anything that impacts upon his future wellbeing. And what do you think is the single most valuable possession that your baby has? What do you think is the single thing that impacts more than anything else on your baby's future wellbeing, happiness and prospects? What is it that the research again and again shows predicts your baby's future, from his intellectual abilities to his psychological stability to his chances at having a happy relationship? If you aren't sure, take a good look in the mirror. The biggest thing your baby has going for him is you. It is therefore absolutely vital for your baby's wellbeing that you take care of yourself.

The purpose of this chapter is to learn how to be kind to yourself. This includes specific exercises for increasing self-kindness. It is essential that mums learn to be kind to themselves. Your needs and your baby's needs are so entwined that in order to fully take care of your baby, you'll need to learn how to take care of yourself.

TAKING CARE OF YOURSELF IS TAKING CARE OF YOUR BABY

The research is very clear. The greatest asset that a baby can have is a mum who loves her and responds to her needs. Loving and supportive parenting predicts a wide range of positive outcomes, from intellectual ability and academic achievement to happiness and self-esteem, to future relationships. All of that loving and supportive parenting takes energy, and is easier and more natural when your own needs are being met. Your baby's most precious possession, her greatest asset, is you. It matters for your baby's long-term future happiness that you are physically, mentally and emotionally as well as you can be. If your baby possessed a precious jewel, wouldn't you take good care of it? In the same way, as her mum, it is vital that you take care of yourself not only for your own good but also for the good of your baby.

It can often seem as if we are forced in the moment to choose between taking care of our baby and taking care of ourselves. For example, an exhausted pregnant woman may need to choose between going to a pilates class and having a much-needed night in, or a new mum may have to choose between giving her hungry baby a feed immediately or taking another minute to finish a sandwich first. However, these choices are not between the baby's self-interest and the mum's self-interest at all, because it is also in the interests of the baby that her mother remains well. In other words, taking care of yourself is taking care of your baby. Conversely, neglecting yourself is neglecting your baby because it involves squandering your baby's greatest treasure. So the exhausted pregnant woman is not choosing between going to a pilates class for her baby or having a night in for herself. In fact she is choosing between the benefits to her baby of her getting some exercise that evening and the benefits to her baby of her having a rest. The real question is, how will each affect her physical, mental and emotional wellbeing and how will that affect her baby? Similarly, the new mum choosing between feeding her hungry baby immediately or finishing a sandwich first isn't choosing between her baby's need for a feed and her own need to eat. Instead she's choosing between her baby's immediate need for a feed and her baby's need for mum to remain physically and emotionally well by getting adequate nutrition and for mum to have enough energy to continue to care for baby for the rest of the day. (And of course, if mum is breastfeeding, that sandwich is also baby's dinner!).

Your baby needs you to remain as well as you can be. So your need for food, rest, sleep, leisure time and social time are all your baby's needs too.

KINDNESS FOR SELF, KINDNESS FOR BABY

In the previous chapter we explored developing and showing kindness towards your baby. In fact, in order to truly show kindness towards your baby it is necessary to also show kindness towards yourself. Women often find it more difficult to develop kindness for themselves than to develop kindness for others. You may not have had a lot of practice in being kind to yourself. Perhaps you may even be in a pattern of bullying yourself, of using force, criticism and 'willpower' to push yourself through the day. Fortunately, being kind to yourself is something at which you can improve with practice. Not only will increased self-kindness support your ability to take care of yourself and hence protect your baby's greatest asset, but also you will be modelling self-kindness for your baby and hence increasing his ability to be kind to himself in the future.

Once learned, self-kindness is the way out of a self-judging, critical relationship to self. When we have a bullying relationship with ourselves and we notice this, we can often try to change this situation by bullying ourselves about that too. For example, we might belittle ourselves for being so stupid as to think that we are stupid all the time. Learning self-kindness is a way out of this vicious cycle.

In the following exercise, you can explicitly practise being kind to yourself. This exercise is suitable for women at all stages, whether you are trying to conceive, pregnant or a new mum. This exercise involves visual imagery and so is best done with your eyes closed.

Self-kindness exercise

Get into a comfortable sitting position, ensuring that you have a straight back but allowing yourself to have a relaxed, comfortable posture. Settle into it. Gently close your eyes. Let your hands rest gently on your knees or in your lap.

Allow your mind to settle gently into the here and now.

Notice the sensations in your body ...

Feelings of touch or pressure where your body makes contact with the floor or the chair ...

Feelings of warmth or cool ...

The rhythm of your breathing ... the gentle in and out.

Notice the sensations as you breathe ...

Use your breath as an anchor to connect to the here and now.

Start to visualise a ball of warm light in your heart ...

This warm light is kindness, compassion, openness.

First, imagine someone whom you naturally feel kindness towards ...
It could be your baby, a good friend, even an animal ...

Let yourself feel kindness towards them, to want the best for them ...

Allow the ball of warm light to grow and radiate out to them, bathing them in kindness ...

Feel yourself open wide to them. If they were here physically, maybe you'd be opening your arms wide and giving them a hug; it is like you are doing that mentally, opening your mind and heart wide open to them exactly as they are.

Now imagine yourself; see yourself standing in front of you ...

Yourself with all your faults, all your weaknesses, all of your history.
As best you can, allow yourself to feel kindness towards yourself ...
Allow the ball of light to grow and radiate out, bathing you in kindness.
Consider that even when you made mistakes, you were searching for
happiness ... See if you can find some kindness for yourself for this.
If you cannot wish for your happiness for your own sake, then wish
for your happiness for the sake of your baby.
Gently open to yourself exactly as you are ...
You may find it helpful to imagine yourself as a baby ...
Imagine that you have travelled back in time and that you are look-
ing at yourself as a newborn baby ...
Didn't that baby need to be loved by an adult exactly as she was?
In that moment, as a newborn baby, weren't you, like all babies, abso-
lutely lovable?
See if you can give your baby self what she needs. You may even like
to imagine giving her a big hug.
Radiate warmth and light towards yourself as a baby ...
Then try to keep radiating warmth and light towards yourself as an
adult, perhaps by watching your baby self grow into your adult self.
If you are feeling stuck, you may like to imagine that you are some-
one who symbolises kindness to you, radiating love towards yourself.
You can imagine that you are a spiritual figure, or a fictional character, or someone that you know.
Feel the ball of light as this person radiates kindness towards you.
When you are ready to end the exercise, do so gently, using your
breathing as an anchor to bring your awareness with you back into
the room. Try to bring this sense of kindness for yourself with you ...

You may find that particular aspects of this exercise are
more helpful in cultivating a sense of kindness towards yourself than others. It is okay to practise this exercise focusing
on the aspects that you find helpful. Being kind to yourself
is a skill like any other, and you will improve with regular
practice. It can be more difficult to be kind to yourself in daily
life, so if you find self-kindness challenging it can be very
beneficial to set aside time each day specifically to practise

cultivating self-kindness. With regular practice, you will find that it becomes easier to do. It will also become easier to be kind to yourself in your daily life.

SELF-KINDNESS IN DAILY LIFE

During our daily lives we might notice at times that we've become locked into a harsh battle with ourselves.

You can use the following suggestions to increase your self-kindness in the moment:

- ✩ Imagine in the future, when your baby has a baby of her own, that they are in exactly the same situation that you are in now. What would you say to them? What would you do? Now try, as best you can, to treat yourself in the same way.

- ✩ Imagine that your best friend was in the same situation that you are now in. What would you say to her? What would you do? Now try, as best you can, to treat yourself in the same way.

- ✩ Imagine that someone you identify as being an example of amazing kindness was with you. It may be someone you know in your real life, a person from fiction, a spiritual figure or even an imaginary person. What would someone with amazing and pure kindness say to you? Try to really absorb their kindness and take it on board.

- ✩ Consider that, like every other human being, you are capable of suffering and happiness. Even when you make mistakes you are just trying, in your own imperfect way, to be happy. See if you can find some kindness in yourself for that.

- ✩ Try to gently wish happiness for yourself. If it seems as if you don't deserve happiness, consider how your happiness would benefit others such as your baby. Doesn't your baby deserve a happy mum?

- ✩ Gently open yourself to your own experience. This doesn't mean that you need to feel any particular way. Rather, it is a stance that you can take towards yourself. If you could express it physically it would be like giving yourself a hug.

✩ Try to hold yourself gently as if you were holding your baby. Feel your grasp on your own experience, thoughts and feelings soften and become gentle.

ACTS OF SELF-KINDNESS

It is also important to *show* kindness towards yourself in your daily life. It may help to first consider some kind acts that you perform, or could do, if another person was having a bad day, and then to think about how you could do similar things for yourself. This could involve simple things like making yourself a cup of tea, taking a short break from baby or having a relaxing night in. If you have a range of ways to show kindness to yourself, then you can draw on these acts when needed.

When you first try being kind to yourself it may feel strange or awkward. Remember that with practice it will feel more natural. If you haven't been kind to yourself much in the past, then being kind to yourself may at first cause your monsters to become very noisy, and it may also trigger feelings of guilt. If this happens, draw on your skills in being mindful of your emotions and thoughts. If being kind to yourself does trigger feelings of guilt and noisy monsters, this is an indication that becoming more kind to yourself may be exactly what you need to be doing. Can you show yourself kindness and accept your noisy monsters as they are— just voices in your head? Continue showing yourself small acts of kindness, and notice what happens with practice.

Think of ways in which you can be kind to yourself:

....

....

....

....

....

....

ACCEPTING OUR MISTAKES

Self-kindness is definitely called for when we make mistakes. All too easily we can become cruel and harsh with ourselves, indulging in self-anger and guilt. Even when we recognise this, we often instinctively try to stop ourselves from bullying ourselves through bullying. Kindness is a way out of this trap. When you make a mistake, hold your thoughts and feelings lightly. Remember that even your mistakes are motivated by just trying to be happy.

While it is helpful to recognise when we have made a mistake so that we can make amends or change our approach in the future, dwelling on the past and on what we've already done is not helpful. Instead of dwelling on the past mistake, think about it in terms of the future. Recognise honestly, and with self-kindness, what you did or did not do that you regret. Next, reconnect with your values in that area. How would you like to have acted, based on your values? Then figure out how you'll change in the future. This may involve changing how you'll handle similar situations next time, or it may be that there is something you can do to remedy the situation now. This is more than simply promising yourself that you'll do things differently next time. Instead, think about how the mistake was made. Are there actions that you could take to lessen the chance that you'll make the mistake again?

For example, if a new mum finds herself yelling at her baby, she won't undo losing her temper by then getting angry with herself or indulging in guilt. Instead, she can recognise that yelling at her baby isn't being the mum that she wants to be. She can start by regretting the action. As feelings of guilt arise she can notice these feelings, make room for them, and let them go. Instead of indulging in guilt, she can focus on the future. The mother can do this by considering how she came to be yelling at her baby. For example, she may realise that she lost her temper because she was looking after her baby by herself during the evening, when her baby is most unsettled, while persisting in trying to get dinner on the table at the same time. She may decide that, in the future, she can try to avoid spending evenings alone with her baby by drawing on support from her partner, family and friends. Further, the mum may decide that if she is alone with her baby and her baby is unsettled, then any housework or cooking will have to wait. She may decide that next time her baby is unsettled she will put on some favourite music and rock her baby in her rocking chair, and if that means having toast for dinner, so be it. In reasoning out how the mistake came to be made, the new mum now has a clear and realistic plan for ensuring that she is not vulnerable to making the same mistake again in the future.

SETTLING BABY, SETTLING SELF

The times when your baby needs settling are likely to be times when you need a bit of kindness too. It is helpful to consider this in building a settling repertoire by using settling techniques that are kind to yourself as well. There are a variety of settling techniques that can be used to settle a baby who is fussing or crying or a baby who needs to go to sleep. Some babies are more difficult to settle than others and all babies will have times when, in spite of a parent's best efforts, they take time to settle. When a baby is taking time to settle, the settling techniques are just as much about settling mum as they are about settling baby.

So it is important that you consider which settling techniques and routines you find soothing and how you can use the settling techniques in a way that soothes you too. For example, you might find particular songs or lullabies soothing, perhaps because you associate the song with positive memories or because you find the nonsensical lyrics amusing. You might find it helpful to set up a particular spot in the house for when baby needs settling, perhaps with a rocking chair and relaxation music at hand. Talking to your baby can also be a wonderful way to settle him too. When your baby is fussing and you are having difficulty settling him, or perhaps you simply cannot respond to him straight away—because you are driving or changing his sister's nappy, for example—talking to your baby is a fantastic way of letting him know that you are still there (even if this doesn't settle him). It is also helpful in taking care of yourself. When you are talking to your baby in this way, try using gentle humour to keep your own mood light; for example, use phrases like, 'Oh dear, the service here is terrible isn't it? Where is that breastfeed?' You can also find phrases that remind yourself of your values; for example, 'Mummy is here for you. Mummy is right here'. In time, specific phrases may become 'mummy mantras' for you—statements that you can say to lighten your mood and remind yourself of why you are pacing the corridor in the middle of the night with a crying baby!

Some popular settling techniques include:

- ✫ offering baby a feed (especially if breastfeeding)
- ✫ offering baby an opportunity to suckle that isn't a feed (such as on your finger or a dummy)
- ✫ rocking baby on a rocking chair
- ✫ trying different holding positions
- ✫ walking with baby
- ✫ singing to baby
- ✫ saying 'shhh'
- ✫ holding baby so baby can hear your heartbeat
- ✫ playing music (lullabies, children's music, relaxation music)
- ✫ playing white noise
- ✫ talking to baby (including using 'mummy mantras')
- ✫ using toys with noises and songs
- ✫ using toys with soft lights
- ✫ having skin-to-skin time
- ✫ changing your scenery (by walking outside or driving the car).

Notice that most of the settling techniques address several of your baby's needs at the same time. For example, taking your baby for a walk outside provides your baby with a change in stimulation as well as an opportunity to settle to sleep if baby is tired and, if you carry your baby for the walk, your baby is able to enjoy physical affection from you as well.

Are there particular baby-settling techniques that you find, or think you'll find, soothing?

....

....

....

....

....

Are there particular phrases or mummy mantras you could say to settle baby that would lighten your own mood or remind you of your values? (Gentle humour can help.)

....

....

....

....

....

As you use the settling techniques, continue to notice which are soothing for you, and build a settling repertoire with consideration not just for what your baby needs but also for what you need. Remember that, even when the settling techniques take time, simply being with your baby when he is unsettled shows your baby that he is loved.

ONE WOMAN'S STORY
Reading Yindi's story may give you ideas on how you can take care of yourself.
Yindi had never been good at being kind to herself. She was good at being kind to everyone else, but not to herself. Yindi usually prioritised the needs of her husband Jarrah, as well as the needs of her family and her friends, over her own needs. She always put

herself last. Yindi was also her own worst critic. Ever since she was a child she had tended to criticise herself harshly, bemoaning every slight 'mistake'. When Yindi fell pregnant, she knew that this had to change. Yindi was used to putting others first and herself second, but she now realised that her baby's needs and her own needs were so entangled that in order to truly put her baby first, she needed to take better care of herself too. Yindi also wanted to stop being so harsh with herself for every mistake, because she didn't want to model that behaviour for her child.

Yindi began to practise the self-kindness exercise daily. She would imagine radiating light and warmth towards herself. At first she found it difficult to feel kindness towards herself. She found it easiest to do so when she imagined herself as a tiny newborn baby. It felt instinctive to feel kind towards a vulnerable baby, even herself as a baby. Gradually, she was able to take this feeling of kindness and keep radiating it towards herself as an adult as well.

As she continued practising the self-kindness exercise daily she found it easier to be kind to herself in her daily life. If she began to be harsh and cruel to herself she would take a deep breath and remember to treat herself with all the gentleness and kindness that she wanted to show to her baby when it was born. Yindi started to deliberately do for herself the sort of kind and considerate things that she regularly did for others. For example, she would make herself her favourite food for dinner or give herself a break by having a night in with a movie. At first it felt strange, but as she kept being kind to herself she found that it became more natural.

As Yindi's pregnancy progressed she was diagnosed with gestational diabetes. Yindi was advised that she needed to make changes in her diet and to do gentle exercise regularly. When she was first diagnosed, Yindi slipped straight into self-blame. She felt consumed with guilt and kept thinking that if only she'd been exercising regularly and eating a healthy diet before falling pregnant she might have escaped gestational diabetes. However, after a day or two of wallowing in self-blame Yindi realised that this wasn't helping. Even if her actions in the past had contributed to her having gestational diabetes, those actions were now done. She had to forgive herself for those mistakes and focus instead on what she could do now to become the mum that she wanted to be.

Yindi found it challenging to change her diet and exercise habits. Every so often she would 'slip' and eat something she wasn't supposed to, go too long between meals or skip exercising. At these times Yindi focused on treating herself kindly. She'd think to herself, 'How would I support a friend in this situation?' Sometimes she would even make time to do her self-kindness exercise. When she was able to be gentle with herself over her slip, she would think through the circumstances leading up to the slip and consider how she could decrease the chances of slipping again. Yindi realised that she was much more likely to slip if she had easy access to junk food or if she was having a busy day. Therefore, to decrease the chances of slipping, Yindi cleared out all of the junk food in her house, and her husband started following the same diet. Jarrah also started cooking more and they would, together, prepare healthy meals and snacks. Yindi started to prioritise having time to herself to relax every day as well as making time to take a walk. In this way, Yindi did the best she could, with gestational diabetes, to be the mum that she wanted to be and to take care of herself at the same time.

MY UNIQUE ADVENTURE
These comments may help you to understand how the information in this chapter might relate to your own unique experiences.

Becoming a confident mum
May be relevant to women at any stage who are struggling to find confidence in their own mothering, coping with self-doubt or coping with criticism and advice from others.
If you are struggling with self-criticism and trying to become more confident, this can become a vicious cycle. You may

catch yourself attacking yourself and, furious with yourself, you attack yourself for that too. Does this sound familiar? It just isn't possible to bully or criticise yourself into confidence. Instead, the vicious cycle of self-criticism needs to be broken with a bit of kindness. If you are highly critical of yourself, practise the self-kindness exercise regularly and try, as best you can, to be kinder to yourself in your everyday life. Remember, it will take practice. Are you becoming kinder to yourself with time?

How do I survive this?

May be relevant to women experiencing emotional challenges, challenging physical symptoms such as morning sickness, or birth. During the most difficult times it is easy to be harsh and critical of ourselves when really it is time for a little self-kindness. Ask yourself, 'If my best friend was experiencing what I'm experiencing right now, how would I help her?' Try to treat yourself in the same way.

Playing the blame game

May be relevant to women at any stage who are caught in the trap of blaming themselves, including where they genuinely have contributed to the situation. Getting caught up in assigning blame for mistakes is a distraction from doing the best you can in the situation that you are now in. Self-flagellation can be tempting, especially if some of your actions genuinely may have led to a negative situation. However, the blame game is a trap. Instead of playing it, start by acknowledging, honestly, what you wish you had done differently. As best you can, do this with kindness. Remember that even when you made mistakes in the past, you were just doing the best you could at the time. Consider if your best friend made the same mistake or if your baby as an adult made the same mistake. What would you tell them?

Next, reconnect with your values. How can you best live out your values in the situation that you are now in? Can you take steps to prevent yourself from making the same mistake again? It is important that you find real actions that you can take here. Don't just try to bully yourself into not making the mistake again, as this won't work. What made you vulnerable to the mistake the first time? Then take whatever steps you can to prevent yourself being vulnerable to making the same mistake again. Remember that your baby will make mistakes too. You are showing your baby what to do when she makes a mistake herself.

PUTTING IT INTO PRACTICE

☆ Notice the times when you are kind to yourself and the times when you are harsh or cruel. Are you able to find kindness for yourself? This isn't about how you feel at the time; rather, it is about showing yourself the same kindness that you might show another in the same situation.

☆ If you think that you could benefit from increased self-kindness then commit to practising the self-kindness exercise regularly, even if just for five minutes a day. It may help to imagine yourself as a baby, or to imagine another person who personifies kindness to you radiating the warm light. Are you able to find kindness for yourself? After practising the exercise regularly for a time, do you notice increased self-kindness in your everyday life?

☆ The next time you make a mistake, notice how you react. Does it benefit anyone to get trapped in guilt or self-recrimination? Try to focus on the future rather than on the past. What contributed to you making the mistake that you did? Are there steps that you can take to decrease the chance that you'll make the same mistake again?

11

Building a rewarding life

The transition to motherhood has flow-on effects for the rest of your life, from the big fixtures of your life such as your working life to the little details, like what you eat for lunch. You will likely find your life changing in pregnancy and then changing again as your baby is born. It is important for our mental health to build a life that is rich in rewards. You may well have built a richly rewarding life before motherhood; however, motherhood has so many flow-on effects that it is probably necessary to rebuild it. In this chapter we explore the importance of building a life that is rich in rewards and examine how to use your values to do so. We also consider what a rewarding life could be for you during pregnancy and in the early months of motherhood.

WHY A REWARDING LIFE IS IMPORTANT

In order to build a rewarding life, it is important that you don't wait until you are in the mood to do so. It is easy to fall into the trap of thinking that you need to be in the right mood first before doing something potentially rewarding, such as joining that mother's group, calling a friend or reading a book. Unfortunately, while you wait for the right mood to strike, you can be living a life that's unfulfilling in the meantime.

Living a life that is rewarding, day by day, aids in stress management and prevents depression. In fact, deliberately increasing daily rewards (as we'll be doing in this chapter) is an evidence-based treatment for depression. Conversely, if you aren't experiencing many rewards day by day then your mood is likely to remain down and sad. In other words, we often think that the mood should come first and then, acting on that mood, we'll do the rewarding activity. In fact, the reverse is true: we need to build a rewarding life first to provide the right environment for happy, positive moods to grow.

VALUES AS GUIDING STARS

Remember the concept of values from Chapter 1? Our values are the things that we deeply care about; those which give our lives meaning and purpose. Although values underpin our goals, they are bigger than goals and can never be fully achieved. Our values matter deeply to us and when we are following them we usually get a strong feeling of satisfaction. Values are long-term desired qualities of living. We can compare our values to guiding stars, as we can use them to lead us through our lives.

In Chapter 1 we explored your values in relation to mothering, but of course you have values in all areas of your life. We can use these values to build a vital, rewarding life. It is helpful to be aware of the values underlying the things that you find gratifying, because this will allow you to be flexible in rebuilding a rewarding life with the changes that occur in the transition to motherhood.

What do you value in your career, job or working life? If you have a job now, what do you find rewarding about your work? If you are currently on maternity leave or have finished work, what did you find rewarding in your job? What qualities do you (or did you) hope to show in your job?

....

....

....

....

....

What do you value in your hobbies and leisure activities? What do you find rewarding about your hobbies and leisure activities? What qualities do you hope to show in your hobbies and leisure activities?

....

....

....

....

....

What do you value in health? What do you find rewarding about health activities or taking care of your health? What qualities do you hope to show in terms of your health?

....

....

....

....

....

What do you value in your social life? What do you find rewarding about social activities or catching up with friends? What qualities do you hope to show in terms of your friendships and social life?

....

....

....

....

....

Do you have religious or spiritual values? If so, what do you find rewarding about your religion or spirituality? What qualities do you hope to show in terms of your religion or spirituality?

....

....

....

....

....

Imagine that you were magically given time that you could spend doing whatever you'd like to do. Every resource you'd need would be magically available and you'd have the energy to pursue your goals. If you could spend time just enjoying yourself this way, what would you do? Why does this matter?

....

....

....

....

....

BUILDING A REWARDING LIFE WHILE TRYING TO CONCEIVE

In order to protect your mental and emotional wellbeing, it is important to ensure that you are living a rewarding life while you are trying to conceive. This is especially important if you are having difficulty conceiving (including if you are using IVF or you are waiting to adopt). It is also important even if you aren't having difficulty. For a healthy couple it may take six to 12 months to conceive, and it is normal to experience emotional highs and lows during this time. You might like to consider whether there any activities that you would enjoy or have always meant to try that you won't be able to do once pregnant. If so, consider trying these activities now to give yourself a special reward during this time of waiting.

You might also like to consider how to build rewards in with your menstrual cycle. If you are still trying to conceive naturally it makes sense to plan rewarding activities during your fertile times that are consistent with conception. For example, your fertile times may be the ideal time to plan for romantic evenings with your partner, for activities together as a couple (for example, taking a walk together), for relaxing activities such as a bath, or to do something that makes you feel special, such as haircuts and beauty treatments. It is obviously beneficial to conception to have an active sex life during your fertile times, but the idea is to do this in a way that makes your fertile time a rewarding and special time for you and your partner rather than a pressure-filled time of stress.

You might like to consider what you'll do when you find out you aren't pregnant or are menstruating. Are there special activities that you could do at that time? You may find it beneficial to build a routine of rewarding activities for this time, such as catching up with a friend or having a long, hot bath.

BUILDING A REWARDING LIFE FOR PREGNANCY

Even if you had a richly rewarding life before pregnancy, falling pregnant may change your lifestyle and you may need to rebuild a rewarding life. During pregnancy, you may find that you need to stop specific activities due to physical symptoms such as morning sickness or exhaustion, or due to medical recommendations, and this may affect your social life. If you experience severe symptoms or complications necessitating bed rest, you may find that your activities are quite restricted and you may need to be creative to ensure that you aren't just lying in bed all day, bored and worried about your baby.

In order to build a rewarding life within the boundaries of your medical recommendations and physical symptoms, use your values. By identifying the values that were underlying your most rewarding activities, you can be more creative and flexible in finding new ways to fulfil these values that are achievable during pregnancy. You may also find that pregnancy is an opportunity to pursue new rewarding activities. Consider activities that are not physically restricted, such as reading, listening to music or surfing the internet, as well as activities that are relaxing and restful, such as meditation. It may be that pregnancy is the perfect time to read books that you've always wanted to read, or to watch a show that you think you'd enjoy.

It is also important to ensure that you continue to have a social life. If you are taking maternity leave, you may be surprised when you finish work how much going to work gave you social contact and structured your life. It is important, therefore, to ensure that your maternity leave while you are waiting for your baby is structured and contains plenty of outings and social activities.

As your due date approaches, you enter a waiting game. It is vital to continue to plan for enjoyable and rewarding activities each day so that you have something to look forward to, even if baby keeps you waiting. Enlist friends and family in keeping you busy at this time.

BUILDING A REWARDING LIFE FOR A NEW MUM

As a new mum it is likely that your lifestyle will have changed in many ways. You may be on maternity leave or have finished work. Your routines for sleeping and eating will change. Leisure and social activities that you previously enjoyed may be impractical, or they may not seem so relevant any more.

Use your values as the basis for rebuilding a rewarding life that includes your new role as a mum. First, consider whether there are ways of pursuing your values (in terms of career, leisure, health or spirituality) in your new role as a mum. For example, values in relation to music may be fulfilled as a mum through singing to your baby. Also consider other activities that, while they aren't part of being a mum, can be fitted into your new lifestyle with baby. For example, if you value health and exercise, you might like to consider the best ways of exercising with your baby. Would you enjoy going for a walk with baby regularly? Or going to an exercise class for new mums? Or following an exercise video while your partner or another support person minds your baby? If your baby's arrival has triggered a change in your working life (that is, if you are taking maternity leave, cutting back your working hours or finishing work), then you might like to consider the values that you were previously fulfilling with your career. There may be other ways of getting the same fulfilment that you used to gain from work. For example, if you find that work is an outlet for your desire to socialise and to meet new people, then it is a good idea to focus on ways that you can socialise as a new mum. If your work gives you intellectual stimulation, then you may need to consider other activities that also give you intellectual stimulation and how you can build these activities into your life as a new mum. If you are taking maternity leave and then returning to work (whether you are returning full time or at reduced hours), you will probably find that you need to adjust to your maternity leave and then adjust again to working and being a mum.

It is important to understand that building a rewarding life is not just about taking 'me time'. If some of your rewarding activities involve a break from baby and you are able to take those breaks, that's fine. If you find that you need regular breaks from your baby anyway, that's fine too and it is quite normal. However, be wary of thinking that anything rewarding for yourself must require a break from your baby. You will quickly find yourself living an unrewarding life! Every mum has limited 'me time', so don't wait for a break to enjoy yourself. Make sure that you are building into your new life plenty of rewarding activities that you can do with your baby too.

As a new mum you will be spending a lot of your time feeding your baby. Especially if you are breastfeeding, this may be a task that is solely yours and there may be times in the day when your baby cluster feeds or feeds for a lengthy period of time. It can be useful to consider activities that you can do while you feed to turn your baby's feeding time into a rewarding and enjoyable break for you. Of course, you may like to have regular feeds where you simply enjoy your baby, perhaps even using the mindfulness of baby exercise to focus on noticing your baby and being present with your baby while you feed. However, you will be feeding your baby six to 12 times a day, or even more, so you will probably not want to do this at every feed. It is useful then to think about activities that you can do when you feed so that feeds are a relaxing break for you.

Some ideas are:

- ☆ recording favourite TV shows and watching them when you feed
- ☆ reading a book or magazine
- ☆ listening to an audiobook
- ☆ listening to a radio podcast
- ☆ watching a movie (a little at every feed throughout a day)
- ☆ surfing the internet or checking emails (for example on a smart phone or tablet computer)
- ☆ feeding outside (such as on your balcony, in your garden or in a park).

SCHEDULING YOUR LIFE

It is vital that you don't wait until you are in the right mood to begin to live a rewarding life. In order to ensure that you aren't tempted to continue to wait, it is useful to plan ahead and schedule rewarding activities. This means opening your diary and looking at the week ahead. What rewarding activities do you have planned? Even small activities such as a relaxing bath can be planned ahead to ensure that they do happen.

Of course, this doesn't mean that you can't also be flexible to fit in with your baby, particularly if you are a new mum. If your baby is feeding frequently or if you've had a particularly poor night's sleep, it may make sense to revise your plans. There is nothing wrong with being flexible and changing your plans, as long as you change your plans to new plans that suit you better. Don't simply cancel your plans. For example, after a night of very little sleep due to your baby feeding frequently, you might change your planned outing with your friends to another day and instead treat yourself to a day of relaxing activities at home.

Don't forget about...

The exact activities that you choose to build into your schedule are unique to you, based on your values and what is enjoyable to you. That said, there are some things that everyone should consider. First, you should consider building into your schedule some kind of physical activity. Regular physical exercise promotes both physical and mental health. When choosing the kind of physical activity that you will undertake, do follow medical advice and consider any current physical symptoms. Gentler types of physical activity, or activities designed specifically for pregnancy or the postpartum period, may be ideal, such as walking, swimming, and pregnancy or postpartum yoga and exercise classes. Also consider your values. If you don't have strong values in relation to physical activity then maybe you can find a way to incorporate other values into your physical exercise. For example, a walk in the park may be ideal if you enjoy the outdoors, or you may enjoy a pregnancy exercise class as an opportunity to socialise with other pregnant mums. Of course, if you are advised to refrain from physical activity by your doctor or midwife then you should follow this advice.

You should also consider building social activities into your schedule. Everyone needs a regular dose of social activity to maintain their mental and emotional wellbeing. As you journey towards motherhood your social life may change dramatically. Going on maternity leave and changes in friendships (particularly if your friends don't have children or have a different parenting style to you) may mean that you need to find new social activities. You may be surprised at how much your working life contributed to your social wellbeing or at how much you may lose interest in social activities that you previously enjoyed. Do ensure that you make contact with friends and family regularly, and begin new social activities if need be.

It is also important for everyone to consider the kinds of activities that, while they aren't necessarily rewarding as such at the time, do give you a boost when they are completed. Activities such as cleaning, ensuring that the fridge is stocked with nice food, having a shower and putting on nice clothes are all activities that may make you feel better during the day. The important point here is that you need to consider how these activities fit with your values. Often, people may tell a new mum simply to leave the cleaning, or that it is a good idea to stay in bed in your pyjamas for the first few weeks. For many women these may be fantastic ideas. If staying in your pyjamas makes you feel comfortable and relaxed, then it is a great idea for you. If, however, staying in your pyjamas makes you feel uncomfortable and down then it makes sense for you to prioritise having a shower and getting dressed in the morning, and to work out how you are going to make that happen. The same goes for cleaning your house. If there are areas of the house that you enjoy being clean, then this should be prioritised and you need to figure out how to achieve it.

Some ideas to keep on top of these activities when baby arrives may include outsourcing (for cleaning); enlisting help from your partner; enlisting help from social support; using swings, bouncers or rockers (for example, try showering with your baby in the bathroom in a swing, bouncer or rocker—just leave the door open so that baby doesn't overheat); taking opportunities during baby's naps; or carrying the baby in a sling/possum pouch while completing some of your household chores, such as dusting. The important point is that the cleaning, self-care and related activities that you prioritise when baby is born should be based on what you find rewarding and revitalising, not on thoughts of what you should do or worries about what other people will think of you.

THINK SMALL–REALLY SMALL

When thinking of activities to build a rewarding life, most people quickly and easily think of bigger things. It is okay to have some bigger activities scheduled into your week, provided that they are realistic. For example, activities like attending an exercise class, seeing a movie with a friend, organising the nursery, doing a 20 minute meditation or gardening are bigger activities. You may be thinking that these activities aren't really that big, but they all require a certain amount of effort and time. It is easy for the physical symptoms of pregnancy, exhaustion from sleep deprivation, a fussy baby or a lack of time to make these plans unrealistic. Even on a good day, there are limitations to how many bigger rewards you can fit into your schedule. Thus, it is also important to think about the small rewards that you can build into your day.

The truly small rewards are things that, while rewarding, require minimum effort or time to do. These activities can realistically be done even with physical symptoms, exhaustion, a fussy baby or a shortage of time. Even though these rewards are small, don't underestimate the value of having many small rewards regularly in your life. It is surprising how big a difference *small* rewards can make.

Some ideas for small rewards include:
- ☆ reading a book or magazine
- ☆ listening to the radio
- ☆ sitting outside
- ☆ calling a friend or family member for a chat
- ☆ eating an enjoyable meal (try planning ahead to have a favourite food available)
- ☆ listening to music
- ☆ singing a favourite song
- ☆ watching a favourite TV show or movie
- ☆ wearing a nice outfit
- ☆ taking a walk
- ☆ spending time with a pet
- ☆ having a cup of coffee or herbal/black tea

- ☆ writing an email or catching up with friends/family using social media
- ☆ looking at photos
- ☆ taking a nap
- ☆ having a relaxing shower or bath.

Remember that the ideas on this list are just ideas. Some of these you may not find very rewarding, or you may not find them to be very easy in your situation. It is best to come up with your own list, based on what is uniquely rewarding for you and what is easy for you to do. When you have thought of some appropriate small activities, consider how you could build these small rewards into your normal day. For example, you could decide to eat your breakfast outside regularly, or to play music every evening, or to ensure that you have some favourite foods in the fridge to make easy and enjoyable lunches. It is also handy to have a rainy day list. The rainy day list includes lots of easy-to-do and small rewards. When you are having a bad day, your rainy day list can help you to plan an enjoyable day in spite of the current obstacles.

BUILDING YOUR REWARDING LIFE

First, look through your values and think up some rewarding activities that you could do based on your values:

....

....

....

....

....

....

Are particular activities realistic at the moment?

....

....

....

....

....

....

Now, think small. Think of some small rewards that you can build into your day. Remember that truly small rewards should be things that require minimum time and effort.

....

....

....

....

....

....

Now that you've done the brainstorming, it is time to open your diary or a calendar and schedule in some of these activities and rewards. You may need to make enquires about some of the activities (such as exercise classes) or you may need to call other people to organise some activities (for example, social activities). If so, start to make these plans. Are there small rewards that you can build into your daily routine?

After you have scheduled in your rewards it is also important to build a rainy day list. Your rainy day list should include lots of small rewards that are easy for you to do.

When I have a bad day I can:

....

....

....

....

....

....

....

Now that you have your schedule and rainy day list, the only thing left to do is to put your plans into action. Remember, it is important to take action now rather than wait until the right mood strikes you, but it is also okay to be flexible. If you find that the plans you made are no longer realistic on a given day, then substitute enjoyable activities from the rainy day list so that you still have a rewarding day.

ONE WOMAN'S STORY
Reading about how Becky built a rewarding life as a mum may help you to apply this in your own life.

Becky kept working right up until she was 39 weeks pregnant. Her baby Oscar arrived by emergency Caesarean two days after she finished work. It was a long labour and Becky found that she spent the first few days in a haze of exhaustion and the next few days weeping with the baby blues. Just as she was beginning to feel normal she was discharged from hospital, and the real challenges began. Becky's husband Alexander worked long hours and didn't take much time off when Oscar was born, so Becky quickly found herself at home alone with the baby. Becky felt like she had been catapulted from one life-style, full-time work, straight into a whole new world. She was shocked at how much time caring for baby Oscar took. Days sped by and all she seemed to do was feed the baby and change his nappies, again and again and again. As each day ended she would despair, feeling as if she'd achieved nothing, and as each day began she would feel exhausted and bleak as if she had nothing to look forward to. She loved baby Oscar but she hated looking after him. Her mood was quickly spiralling downwards with every day. She knew she had to make some changes.

Looking at her life as a new mum, she realised that it just wasn't rewarding. Before Oscar was born, Becky's job had provided structure to her life and many rewards. Becky had enjoyed socialising at work and had loved the sense of achievement as she completed tasks throughout her working day. There had even been many little rewards that she no longer received, such as dressing well, a nice cup of coffee in the morning, the walks to and from the train station to go into work, listening to music during the train ride and tasty lunches. She realised that she needed to provide structure in her life and to ensure that her life was rewarding again.

First, Becky made some decisions about which rewards to build into her daily routine. She decided that she needed to prioritise having a shower and getting dressed in the morning, and that she would wear a nice outfit even if she was just staying at home. She felt better if she was nicely dressed. Becky also decided that during feeds she would either watch TV or listen to an audiobook (borrowed from the library). She also began to have a walk to the local park with baby Oscar every afternoon, as she enjoyed getting fresh air.

Next, Becky decided to write a list each day of tasks that she wanted to achieve; for example housework, activities with Oscar such as bathing him or reading him a story, and outings such as catching up with friends. Ticking off each task as it was completed gave Becky a sense of achievement, and she realised that she really was achieving a lot every day. Every few days she'd plan a bigger rewarding activity, like catching up with her sister, attending a local mother's group or having lunch with a friend. Importantly, she knew that she couldn't wait until she felt like it. She knew that she needed to build a rewarding life first, and then her mood would improve. And on the bad days she always had her rainy day list. Her favourite small act was to simply put on her favourite music. She could do this no matter what was happening with baby Oscar, and slowly but surely, as she sang along, she would feel better.

MY UNIQUE ADVENTURE

These comments may help you to understand how the information in this chapter might relate to your own unique experiences.

Adoption

May be relevant to mums waiting to adopt or new mums of adopted babies.

New mums of adopted babies play a waiting game too—waiting for their own baby to arrive. Ensure that you build yourself a rewarding life while you are waiting. Are there activities that you know you won't be able to do as a new mum that you could do now while you wait? When your new baby arrives you will also need to rebuild a rewarding life as a new mum.

Reversing the downward spiral

May be relevant to women with a history of depression, at risk of postnatal depression or experiencing postnatal depression.

Building a rewarding life is vital to preventing and recovering from depression. If you have a history of depression or are experiencing postnatal depression, it is important that you ensure that your life is full of rewarding experiences. The most important lesson is that you build the rewarding life first and experience the positive mood later. In other words, don't wait until you are in the mood for the rewarding activities. In order to ensure that you stick to living a rewarding life even before you feel like it, it is often helpful to schedule the activities in using a diary or a calendar. You can even schedule in smaller activities like having a relaxing bath. When you plan out your rewarding life in advance it is easier to stick to it.

How do I survive this?

May be relevant to women experiencing emotional challenges, challenging physical symptoms such as morning sickness, or birth.

The challenging times are times for your rainy day list. Pick out some small rewards that are truly easy to do in your current circumstances and use them. Don't be surprised if you don't notice an immediate effect or if the rewards are less enjoyable than usual. When you are coping with a physical challenge such as severe morning sickness, you may find that everything is less enjoyable. However, it is still important to ensure that you are experiencing a rewarding life in order to prevent depression. It may take some creativity to find the best way of building rewards into your life at present, but it is important to do.

Young mums and unplanned pregnancies
May be relevant to young mothers, younger-than-planned mothers and women experiencing an unplanned pregnancy.

If you are a young mum, you may feel that you didn't have the opportunity to build a rewarding adult life before becoming a mother. You may find that completing education, finding a satisfying working life, cultivating adult friendships, increasing independence from your own parents and finding a long-term romantic partner are tasks that are still in your future. It is important to recognise that it is still important for you to have the opportunity to build a rewarding adult life for yourself. This is important not just for your own happiness but also in order to take care of yourself into the future so that you can take care of your baby. You may find it helpful to connect with other young mums. You may also find it helpful to discuss how you are going to build a rewarding life as a new mum and how you are going to continue to build a rewarding adult life with your main support people.

PUTTING IT INTO PRACTICE
- ☆ Are you currently living a rewarding life? If you are pregnant or a new mum, think about how your life has changed so far. Has this led to a decrease in rewards? Has it led to a decrease in a particular type of rewards such as social contact or intellectual stimulation?
- ☆ Schedule rewarding activities into your coming week and plan how you will build small rewards into your daily routine. Remember that it is important to start building rewards into

your life even if you don't yet feel like it. Are there times when you don't feel like doing a planned rewarding activity, but when you do it anyway, you find that you enjoy it? Notice the effects of building small rewards into your daily routine. Often really small rewards, such as dressing nicely or eating a favourite lunch, can have surprisingly big effects on our mood.

☆ Write a rainy day list and put it somewhere where you can easily see it on your bad days. The next time you have a bad day, go to your rainy day list and pick a small reward. Notice the effects of this.

12

Social
support

Having reliable and helpful support from friends and family, both practical and emotional, makes the transition to motherhood much easier. However, the transition to motherhood itself can often create changes in our social world. Our family takes on a new role in our life in relation to our new baby, and friendships may become closer or more distant as our own priorities change. Furthermore, pre-existing difficulties in our friendships or family relationships can become more obvious.

In spite of how important social support is, it is not uncommon to experience challenges in receiving enough and the right kind of support. The purpose of this chapter is to examine how you can maximise the social support that you have in a way that is consistent with your values in relation to family and friends. This includes examining how to handle common difficulties in accessing social support.

MY VALUES IN RELATION TO FAMILY AND FRIENDSHIPS
Let's begin by examining your unique values in relation to family and friendships. Remember that your values are there to guide you. It is important that all women feel supported during the transition to motherhood, but different women

will value different kinds of support, different relationships with family and in-laws and different kinds of friendships, and will enjoy different ways of socialising. This is about you being able to access the support that you need in a way that you enjoy.

What do you *value* in your family life (and your in-law family life if relevant)? What do you find rewarding in your roles as a daughter, sister or aunt? What qualities do you hope to show in family roles?

....

....

....

....

....

....

What do you *enjoy* in your family life? How would you like to share your journey to motherhood with your family? How would you like your baby to fit into your family?

....

....

....

....

....

....

What do you value in your life with friends? What do you find rewarding in your role as a friend? What qualities do you hope to show in your friendships?

....

....

....

....

....

....

....

What do you enjoy in your friendships and social activities? How would you like to share your journey to motherhood with your friends? How would you like your baby to fit into your friendships?

....

....

....

....

....

....

What do you value in your wider social life, for example your relationships with work colleagues, neighbours, or fellow members of religious or community groups? What qualities do you hope to show in your wider social life? What do you find rewarding?

....

....

....

....

....

....

What do you enjoy in your wider social life? How would you like to share your journey with your wider social community? How would you like your baby to fit into your wider community?

....

....

....

....

....

....

These values will form the foundation for how your life within your family, friendship circle and wider community continues once you become a mum.

SURVEYING MY SOCIAL WORLD

The next step is to survey what your social world is currently like and how it may change during your transition to motherhood. First, consider your family. What are your relationships with your family currently like? How are your relationships likely to change throughout pregnancy and after your baby is born? Remember that your family members also have their own relationships to your new baby, and as you become a mum they'll become grandparents or aunts and uncles.

What roles might family members play in your baby's life?

....

....

....

....

....

....

Next, consider friendships. What are your friendships currently like? How might your friendships change throughout pregnancy and after your baby is born? How do you currently socialise with friends? Does that fit with being a mum?

Do you think your friends might play a role in your baby's life? If so, how?

....

....

....

....

....

....

....

Finally, consider your wider social community, including members of your local community, fellow members of sport or exercise groups or friends of friends. What are your relationships in the wider community currently like? How are these relationships likely to change throughout pregnancy and after your baby is born? How do you currently socialise in your wider community? Does that fit with being a mum?

Do you think that people in your wider community have a role to play in your baby's life? If so, how?

....

....

....

....

....

....

....

Now think about what this means in terms of your social support. There are two kinds of social support, and both are important. The first type is emotional support. People in your life who provide emotional support are people to whom you can talk about any difficulties that you are having; people who show understanding and boost your confidence as well as people who support you by just 'being there'. The second type is practical support. Practical support is all of the concrete, doing ways of giving support. It includes people helping out with the housework, cooking you a meal, driving you to an appointment, mowing your lawn, babysitting, or helping you to put together the nursery.

Who is currently providing you with emotional support?

....

....

....

....

....

....

Are there others in your life who could provide you with emotional support if needed? For example, are there friends with whom you could reconnect, or family members who would be good listeners if you did need to talk to them?

....

....

....

....

....

....

....

Who is currently providing you with practical support?

....

....

....

....

....

....

Are there others in your life who could provide practical support? For example, are there friends who would happily help
you set up the nursery if you asked, or family members who
could cook you a meal if you let them know that this would
be helpful?

....

....

....

....

....

....

Do you have enough emotional and practical support? Do
you have back-up options that you could draw upon if needed?
Do you have any difficulties in accessing your support?

....

....

....

....

....

....

We will return later to look at solutions to some common difficulties that people have in accessing social support. First, though, let's examine how to have positive relationships with others in a more broad sense.

BUILDING POSITIVE RELATIONSHIPS

It is important for our own wellbeing and for the quality of our relationships with family, friends and others in our community that we are realistic. Being realistic in our relationships begins with the realisation that we can't control what other people do. That may seem very simple, but it is so easy to forget that I'll say it again: we can't control what other people do. We can only control what *we* do. Building a positive relationship requires positive actions on the part of both people involved in the relationship. So, building a close relationship with your parents requires action on your part and it requires action on their part. Maintaining a strong friendship with your best friend requires action from you and action from her as well. As we cannot control what other people do we cannot ensure that we build a positive relationship. All we can do is to fulfil our side of the bargain, to put in the actions necessary from our end and to act in accordance with our values. What the other person chooses to do is then up to them.

The second aspect of being realistic in our relationships is about accepting that the people in our lives are who they are. The best predictor of future behaviour is past behaviour. If a family member or a friend has acted a certain way for years in their relationship with you—for example, if they are critical, a terrible listener or bad at making contact—then there's a good chance that they are going to continue acting that way. Accepting that people in our lives are who they are doesn't mean that you need to like how they behave, or that they are right, or that you need to put up with their behaviour. It just means that you accept that this is what they do. With realistic expectations of them you can then decide what you are going to do, based on your values.

When we have a more realistic view of the people in our lives, this can help us to draw from them the support that is available. You may well, for example, have someone in your family who is terrible at providing emotional support but who may be ready and willing to provide practical support. Instead of struggling to turn this family member into a good listener, why not accept that they are who they are and make the most of their practical support instead?

With a realistic view of others, you can choose how you want to be in your relationships. Of course, this should be influenced by your unique values. However, we should all consider using effective communication strategies and rewarding the other person when they do something that we do like, because these ways of interacting with other people aid in building positive relationships.

EFFECTIVE COMMUNICATION

Effective communication is communication that is assertive. Some people think that assertiveness is about adamantly standing your ground or being stubborn. In fact, assertiveness is a style of communicating with others that is direct, honest and respectful. There are simple ways to begin to make your style of communicating more assertive, and we'll go through these shortly.

First, though, it is important to understand that assertiveness actually involves far more than just the style of communication. In fact, the heart of assertiveness is accepting yourself as you are and accepting the other person as they are, and working towards fulfilling both of your needs as best you can. An aggressive stance towards others is focused on getting one's own needs met at the expense of the other. An aggressive stance is uncaring and unkind towards others. Conversely, a passive stance towards others is focused on fulfilling the others needs at the expense of the self. A passive stance is uncaring and unkind towards oneself. An assertive stance, on the other hand, is the balance of these two extremes as it involves trying to meet both needs and is caring and kind towards both the other and the self.

Trying to learn an assertive communication style by rote before building self-acceptance and self-kindness may not lead to true assertiveness in your everyday life. In addition, it is possible to use an assertive communication style but to still be using it selfishly. Neither of these is true assertiveness. To be assertive it isn't always necessary to use any of the tips below for assertive communication, and they should be seen as useful pointers only. Instead of just adopting an assertive style when you communicate, try also to build your relationships on acceptance of yourself and the other person.

Expressing yourself assertively also isn't just about what you say and how you say it. It is equally about what you know you don't have to say. In other words, it is about knowing that you don't need to justify or explain yourself. You have every right to say no to an invitation without any need to explain your response. You also have every right to mother the way you want to mother without the need to explain your actions or to justify yourself.

Finally, assertive communication is also not just about how you express yourself; it is also about how well you listen to others.

Try these tips for a more assertive style of communication:

- ☆ Use 'I' statements rather than 'you' statements; for example, 'I'm feeling bombarded here' rather than, 'you're always telling me what to do'.
- ☆ Use factual descriptions rather than judgments or exaggerations; for example, 'I've noticed that you give Alex back to me when she starts to cry' rather than, 'You're hopeless at settling Alex'.
- ☆ Express thoughts, feelings and opinions reflecting ownership; for example, 'I feel it is important that Olivia receives plenty of physical affection' rather than, 'Everyone should cuddle their baby! Are you insane?'
- ☆ Use clear, direct requests or directives when you want others to do something rather than hinting, being indirect or

presuming; for example, 'Can you please pick up a loaf of bread on your way over?' rather than, 'Um . . . I'm not sure what we can have for lunch . . . ah . . . '

☆ Say 'no' politely and firmly to requests that you want to refuse; for example, 'No, thanks. I'm taking it easy this week' rather than, 'Oh, I'd love to but I can't because . . . um . . . I'll be busy that day . . . '

☆ Be realistic, respectful and honest; for example, 'I'm avoiding cigarette smoke during pregnancy so I need you to take that outside,' rather than, 'Yuck! I don't want filthy smoke in my house. How could you do that to my baby?'

☆ Express your feelings honestly; for example, 'Honestly, I'm feeling really disappointed that we're cancelling tonight', rather than, 'Oh no, that's okay, it doesn't bother me at all' (when it does in fact disappoint you).

☆ Use minimal encouragers to show that you are listening. A minimal encourager is a simple way of showing interest without disrupting the speaker's flow. It can be verbal or non-verbal; for example, nodding, 'uh-huh', 'yes', 'I see', 'mmm'.

☆ Paraphrase the information or thoughts that the speaker expressed to you. This shows the speaker that you're listening and that you understand what they said. It can also be used to check that you understand the speaker's message; for example, 'It sounds like you're worried you won't see baby enough?'

☆ Acknowledge the speaker's feelings. If the speaker has said what they are feeling it is important to paraphrase this. If the speaker hasn't said what they are feeling you can trust your intuition, make a guess and put their feelings into words. This demonstrates your empathy. It can also be used to check that you've correctly deduced the speaker's feelings; for example, 'You're feeling pretty angry about this'.

IGNORE THE BAD AND REWARD THE GOOD

You cannot control how others behave, but you can encourage more of the behaviour that you'd like to see by rewarding it when it happens. Ignoring the behaviour we don't like and rewarding the behaviour we do is the most powerful way that we can encourage others to change. Unfortunately, however, this sensible approach is often the reverse of what we actually do! Instead, we usually complain and gripe when someone does what we don't want, and we take it for granted when they behave as we want them to. We can also make things worse by being critical of the person just when they are beginning to change their behaviour by trying to do something we'd like them to do. For example, if you'd like the grandparents to be able to settle your baby, then you'll need to be supportive of them when they try to do so. This doesn't mean that you can't share with them the ways of settling that you've found to be effective, but it does mean that you need to hold off on the criticism and give them the space to find the settling techniques that work for them. Remember that even if they have a lot of experience with babies, they'll still need to find what works for them with *your* baby.

The bottom line is that when someone makes a step in the right direction, even if it is only a small one, or later than you wanted, or imperfectly executed, you still need to encourage them if you want them to take another step next time.

IMPROVING SOCIAL SUPPORT

Let's return to improving your social support. Look back at your survey of your social world. Do you have enough social support? Or perhaps you have enough but you have difficulties in accessing it, or in accessing the right kinds of support? There are four key difficulties that women may have in accessing social support in the transition to motherhood. Many women may experience a combination of these four difficulties, which are:

1 There just isn't enough support.
2 My own thoughts and feelings stop me from asking for or using the support that is available.
3 I don't know how to communicate what I need.

4 My support people give advice or do things that contradict my values.

Let's examine each of these difficulties in turn.

There just isn't enough support

If you and your partner don't have close relationships with your families, or if your families don't live close by or cannot help out for some reason, it is easy to find yourself without a lot of support. You can also find yourself without enough support if you have fallen pregnant at a time when most of your friends are not yet considering having children.

It may be that only one of the types of support is missing, so you may have plenty of emotional support but not enough practical support, for example. Or sometimes it is the right kind of emotional support that is missing. If you've experienced a specific event in the journey to motherhood such as a miscarriage, stillbirth, preterm birth or the birth of a baby with a disability, you may find that your family and friends don't understand the specific challenges that you are facing.

Regardless of why you have insufficient support, there is really only one solution to your problem and that is to seek out further sources of support. Fortunately, you are not the only woman in this position, and seeking connections with other women who are also pregnant or are new mums is a fantastic way of building a strong support network. If you need support from others who understand the specific challenges that you are facing, then seek assistance from parent support organisations in relation to that particular experience; for example, parent support organisations exist for prematurity and for parents of children with specific disabilities. If you are unsure of what support is available in a specific area, discuss this with your doctor, midwife or maternity and child health nurse.

Here are some ideas for connecting with other mums:

☆ Discuss your support needs with your midwife, doctor or maternity and child health nurse and ask them to put you in touch with support groups in your local area or with groups that provide support for specific challenges.

☆ Seek out mothers groups in your area through the internet, word of mouth or specific support groups.

☆ Connect with mothers within your wider community, such as neighbours, friends of friends, fellow members of community or religious organisations, fellow members of sporting or exercises groups, members of your local community and workmates.

☆ Connect with other mums on web-based support groups and forums.

It is also possible that there are other sources of support waiting to be accessed. You may need to look to your wider community for support. If a workmate, a friend of a friend, a neighbour or a distant relative offers to help if you need it, why not take them up on the offer? Anytime someone says that you can give them a call if you need it, write that person's number down and when you need something, call them. Often we don't access support from people more removed from us because we feel uncomfortable. However, when people offer assistance it is usually sincerely meant. Most times when people support others they themselves feel good, and often such times are opportunities to build a closer and mutually beneficial relationship.

If you feel that friends and family members don't understand the specific challenges that you are facing, try using assertive communication skills to clearly explain to them what you are experiencing and how they can support you. Sometimes people may not understand the challenges that another person is facing simply through ignorance, whereas they will be ready and willing to offer the right kinds of support once they do understand.

If your personal support network is lacking then it is particularly important to make the most of the health professionals who are available to support you.

You may like to consider:

- ☆ openly discussing your support needs with your midwife, doctor or maternity and child health nurse and finding out what support can be provided within the healthcare system
- ☆ openly discussing your emotional needs with your midwife, doctor or maternity and child health nurse regularly so that they have the opportunity in their consultation to provide you with whatever support they can (even if this is simply being told that you are doing a fantastic job)
- ☆ connecting with a student midwife who needs to follow a pregnancy as part of their studies. Discuss this with your midwife or doctor, or try phoning the nursing school at local universities.

If you lack practical support, you may be able to make up for this through outsourcing or by scaling back your housework.

If sources of practical support are limited, you may consider:

- ☆ outsourcing housework and/or yard work
- ☆ ordering groceries online
- ☆ using a company that delivers readymade meals
- ☆ scaling back housework, such as by using disposable nappies to cut back on the laundry.

My own thoughts and feelings stop me from asking for or using support that is available

Even when support is readily available, our monsters often show up as we try to access it, and sometimes we can allow our thoughts and feelings to stop us from using potential sources of support. For example, the *I must be a perfect mum* monster may show up and tell you that you have to do all of your housework yourself and to a perfect standard, or else you aren't doing a good enough job. If you allow yourself to believe this story then you may not access available practical support from your family and friends. *The I'm not a good enough mum* monster may tell you that every other mum is coping and that it is just you who is struggling with breastfeeding or sleeping difficulties or crying. If you believe this story then you may not share your struggles with other mums, and you may miss out not only on their emotional support but also the discovery that they too are having similar difficulties (not to mention missing out on being able to brainstorm ways of coping together).

Are your thoughts and feelings getting in the way of accessing support? If so, what are the kinds of stories that you are buying into that are keeping you from accessing your support?

....

....

....

....

....

....

Are there particular emotions that are getting in the way of accessing support? For example, would you feel guilty if you accessed support?

....

....

....

....

....

....

How can you use the skills in this book to allow the monsters to be there and to still access support? Do you need to apply skills to remember that thoughts are just thoughts, or to accept emotions?

....

....

....

....

....

....

I don't know how to communicate what I need

This difficulty calls for you to develop greater assertiveness in your communication. Remember that assertiveness is based on acknowledging both your own needs and the needs of the other person. What kinds of support do you need? What are the needs of your family and friends?

Sometimes we can misjudge the needs of the people closest to us. Particularly during the transition to motherhood, our family and friends may in fact need and want to give us support. Remember that just as you are becoming a mum, your family members are becoming grandparents and aunts and uncles. Your friends, too, may enjoy the opportunity to offer support. Try opening up an honest discussion with them so that you can know their true desires.

You might like to open up discussion with a question:

- ✩ 'How often would you like to see baby when he or she is born?'
- ✩ 'Are you keen to help out with babysitting?'
- ✩ 'How do you feel about doing things like nappy changing?'
- ✩ 'Would you like to come to one of my midwife/obstetrician appointments with me?'

Once you have a clearer view of their needs, you may well find that they want to find ways to support you too. Use your assertiveness skills to communicate your needs for support. Say what you need honestly, openly and respectfully—and above all, just say it! Remember that communicating your needs for support in a relationship usually makes the other person feel special and valued, not burdened.

Try the following statements:

- ✩ 'Something that would be really helpful is if you could cook us a meal or help out with the housework.'

☆ 'I'd love for baby to be close to you, so if you are keen to do some babysitting just say so. It would really help me out as well.'

☆ 'I'd love for you to be there at my next midwife/obstetrician appointment.'

There may be more support available in your wider community than you realise if you are able to communicate your needs assertively. You may find it useful to think through the needs of the person with whom you are communicating and show that you understand their perspective. For example, when communicating to your boss at work your needs for greater flexibility during the months of morning sickness, or for a private space to express breast milk after returning to work, you may find it helpful to start the conversation by talking about how much you value your work and think it is important to be able to be as efficient and productive as possible during your working hours. Explain how the increased flexibility or lactation space will help you to meet your boss's expectations better.

My support people give advice or do things that contradict my values

First of all, remember that you are your baby's mother. No matter what role anyone else plays in your baby's life, and no matter how they choose to play their roles, your baby has only one mum, and it is you. You, and only you, determine the kind of mum your baby has. Only you have control over how you mother your baby. Not only does no one in your baby's life have the right to take this away from you, they can't. There is also no need to justify your mothering decisions to others; they are yours and yours alone. You have every right to be the kind of mum that you want to be. There are also wider parenting decisions that may need to be negotiated between yourself and your baby's father, but again these decisions belong to the two of you and you don't need to justify your approach to others.

We also need to distinguish between the actions that a support person may take and the advice they may give. Let's start with advice. It is not uncommon during the transition to motherhood to be given advice that contradicts your own approach, doesn't work with your unique baby or in your circumstances, is out of date or is, quite frankly, mad. Remember that guidelines on many aspects of pregnancy, health and babycare have changed dramatically over the past 20 to 30 years. Sometimes older relatives are simply passing onto you what was, when they were parenting, the standard parenting or medical advice. And often they are simply telling you what they did with their own children.

It is also important to remember that different people have different values and are parenting in different circumstances. Sometimes a support person's advice makes sense for them because it fits with their values and suits their circumstances. But that doesn't mean that it makes sense for you! Sometimes a gentle reminder that everyone is different can do wonders.

Ultimately, unhelpful advice doesn't require any action at all. Again, remember that you are your baby's mum, and advice is just talk. Your mothering decisions are yours alone, so you don't need to justify yourself. And as you don't need to justify yourself, it is often unnecessary to launch into an explanation of why you won't be acting on the advice, or what your approach will be and why. It certainly isn't necessary to debate your approach, so don't be drawn into an argument (unless it would be a friendly debate that you'd enjoy, in which case go ahead). Remember, you are not obligated to negotiate your approach with anyone who offers you advice. The mothering decisions are yours to make.

Try these responses to advice contradicting your approach:
✩ 'I'll keep that in mind.'
✩ 'That's an interesting idea.'
✩ 'That worked well for you huh? Well, that's great.'
✩ 'Nice to know that worked for your baby. I'm finding that .... works for my baby.'
✩ 'Babies are so different! It is amazing how .... worked so well for your baby and .... works so well for mine.'

☆ 'We're doing .... and it is working well for us.'

If people criticise your approach or make doom and gloom predictions about how your approach will affect your baby, try a matter-of-fact response or even using gentle humour to diffuse the situation and avoid being drawn into a debate.

Try some of these responses:

☆ 'Oh, I'm planning on spoiling her.'

☆ 'We're not worried about that.'

☆ 'Works for us!'

☆ 'That doesn't bother me.'

☆ 'Yeah, he's got me wrapped around his little finger.'

☆ 'That's how we roll in this house.'

In contrast, the actions that a support person may take often do require assertive communication on your part. As the mother, it is your role (along with your baby's father or co-parent if relevant) to place boundaries for others in terms of your baby's health and safety, to make overarching decisions about how your baby will be raised and to advocate on behalf of your baby to your family, friends and the wider community. On the other hand, there is also an extent to which the relationship between your baby and other people is the business of these other people. Just as you are your baby's mum, your baby's grandparents are your baby's grandparents, not you! They and they alone can determine how they grandparent, and they need to find ways to be the grandparents that your baby needs that are consistent with their values as grandparents. So there may be times where it is okay for them to take a different approach to you or to do something that you think is less than ideal.

You may find that these issues are particularly challenging if you are relying upon support people for regular child care (because if you are present usually you can simply step in and do what you'd like to see done!).

When communicating with your support people you may find it helpful to try the following:

☆ Communicate on the level of values while being as flexible as you can about how exactly your support people do what you'd like to see done; for example, 'She'll need help to go down for her nap and we don't want her to be left to cry, but I know you'll need to find your own way to help her to sleep and we're happy for you to try lots of different things, like lying down with her, rocking her or putting her in her pram'.

✩ Communicate in a way that shows that the decision has already been made; for example, 'I will give you a bottle of expressed breast milk every day for you to give to him at lunchtime'.

✩ Show that you respect their values at the same time as wanting to live your own; for example, 'I can certainly see how that worked really well for you. Good for you! It doesn't work well for us though.'

✩ Share your feelings, step away from any debate on the 'correct' way to do things and make a personal request; for example, 'It is tough for me to be away from her and if I know that you have her in the possum pouch for a couple of hours every day then it means I can relax and focus on my work'.

✩ Become a broken record, repeating your request assertively, calmly and respectfully until they do as you ask; for example, 'We don't drink hot drinks and cuddle Michael at the same time. I'll take him while you finish your tea . . . I'll take him . . . I'll hold him for now . . . '.

ONE WOMAN'S STORY
Reading Yasmin's story may help you in building your own social support.

Yasmin and Jason knew that with a 20 month old toddler, Charlotte, and a new baby, Miah, they needed more support for their growing family. At first, they weren't entirely sure where to get it. Yasmin's parents live overseas and so, while they were very excited to have a new granddaughter, they couldn't provide much in the way of ongoing practical support. Jason's family lived nearby and were keen to provide more practical support; however, Yasmin and Jason felt that they had very different ideas about parenting. They found them to be critical of their way of doing things. Also, Yasmin's closest friends hadn't yet had children and were focused on their careers and hobbies. They just didn't seem to understand Yasmin's priorities as a mother.

Yasmin and Jason decided to accept from Jason's family the practical support that they were keen to give. Yasmin decided to politely acknowledge the unhelpful advice. She soon developed a routine of Jason's parents visiting once a week with a cooked meal. While Charlotte and baby Miah were minded by their grandparents, Yasmin busied herself with housework. At some point in the visit Jason's mum would make a remark that would make Yasmin bristle. For example, Jason's mum disapproved of Miah's habit of breastfeeding to sleep and often told Yasmin that she should be teaching the baby to fall asleep by herself in her cot instead.

One week, when Jason's mum arrived to find Miah enjoying a nap in Yasmin's arms after being breastfed to sleep, she remarked, 'That baby has you wrapped around her little finger!' Yasmin just laughed and replied, 'Yes, she does!' Yasmin could use humour to move past her mother-in-law's criticism because she knew that Miah had only one mum, and it was her. Yasmin felt it was unnecessary and unhelpful to get into a debate about breastfeeding to sleep. She just recognised that Jason's parents are who they are and accepted the support she was offered by them.

At times, Yasmin needed to use assertive communication with her mother-in-law too. For example, her mother-in-law arrived one week with puréed vegetables and rice cereal and announced that baby Miah was going to have her first taste of solid food. Yasmin matter-of-factly stated that they were not going to introduce solids for at least another month. When her mother-in-law tutted and said that she introduced solids to Jason at that age, Yasmin calmly replied, 'I'm glad that worked for you and Jason. Miah and I are going to wait.'

Yasmin also sought additional emotional support. She decided to join a local mother's group in order to have time with other new mums. She found it really helpful to connect with other women who were experiencing the same kinds of challenges. Each week she'd come along to the group and share her latest challenges, like baby Miah's grisly moments or Charlotte's temper tantrums, only to find that the other mums were experiencing exactly the same challenges with their children. It reminded Yasmin that the challenges she was experiencing were all normal. Yasmin also decided to be proactive and to reconnect with friends and family with whom she'd lost touch over the years and who might be supportive. She was able to reconnect with an old friend who had two children herself, and so understood Yasmin's current situation and found her a wealth of emotional support and helpful advice.

MY UNIQUE ADVENTURE
These comments may help you to understand how the information in this chapter might relate to your unique experience.

Becoming a confident mum
May be relevant to women at any stage who are struggling to find confidence in their own mothering, coping with self-doubt or coping with criticism and advice from others.
If you want to hear a lot of advice and criticism from other people, become a mum! Unfortunately, other people's advice, even if kindly meant, can be unhelpful in building a new mum's confidence. You may find it liberating to realise that you don't need to justify your approach to others. No matter what the opinions of others are, you are your baby's mum and you alone decide the kind of mum that your baby has. Assertive communication is a skill and it takes practice. Practise being assertive and experiment with responding to advice and criticism until you find ways of responding that work for you.

Help! This wasn't what I had planned!

May be relevant to women experiencing difficulty conceiving, miscarriage, complications, preterm birth, an unwanted birth experience or finding motherhood different from expectations.

If an experience wasn't what we had planned, then it probably wasn't in the plans of the people around us either. You may find yourself in need of support from others who may be willing to give it but may genuinely not understand your needs. It is vital to use assertive communication to clearly explain to others what you are experiencing and what you need from them. Remember if you are experiencing a challenge that your support people have never experienced, they may honestly not realise what it is like for you—not out of any lack of kindness, but from genuine ignorance. With honest and open communication, they may be able to be there for you. It can also be important to connect with people who do understand what you are experiencing because they have experienced the same challenge. You may consider accessing support groups or seeking out other women in the same situation as you in order to share emotional support.

How do I survive this?

May be relevant to women experiencing emotional challenges, tough physical symptoms such as morning sickness, or birth.

If you are experiencing a challenging time, it is vital to fully access your social support, both emotional and practical. Ensure that you are making full use of the social supports that you already have, and use your assertiveness skills to clearly communicate to others what you need. If you need to build additional social support, then seek out other mums or build stronger connections with the family or friends in your own life.

Young mums and unplanned pregnancies

May be relevant to young mothers, younger-than-planned mothers and women experiencing an unplanned pregnancy.

If you are a young mum or if you are experiencing an unplanned pregnancy, your family may be a valuable source of support.

If your pregnancy was unplanned, the father of your baby may not be involved or you may not be in an ongoing relationship with him. In these circumstances it would be normal for other support people, such as your own parents, to play a bigger role in your baby's life and in supporting you. If so, it may be even more important for you to be clear on your own values as a mum and for you to communicate clearly and assertively with your main support people.

If your own parents (or other family members) are going to be heavily involved in supporting you as a mother and in caring for your baby, it is a good idea to discuss with them your values as a mum, their own values as grandparents and what you all feel would be the best roles that you could play in your baby's life. As best you can, be open, honest and assertive.

In addition, you may also find that your friendships change. Consider connecting with other mums or other young mums and building new friendships. Consider also maintaining existing friendships by being as open and honest as you can about your new life. You may also find that it is important for you to regularly have a break from your baby and an opportunity to socialise with your friends, baby-free. You may like to discuss with your support people how to achieve this. Remember, if you are a young mum, it is important for your baby that you still have the opportunity to develop adult friendships and find a long-term romantic partner.

PUTTING IT INTO PRACTICE

✩ Take an inventory of your current social support. Do you need to build up more support? Do you particularly need practical or emotional support? Think through your options for increasing your levels of social support and start taking steps towards this goal. Consider connecting with other new mums through mother's groups or online support, and developing stronger connections with friends or family who may be supportive.

☆ Assertive communication is a skill and, as with any skill, you will improve with practice. Make an effort to begin to communicate more assertively about issues relating to mothering and your baby, as well as about other issues. If you aren't used to communicating assertively, it can sometimes help to try it initially with a stranger in a retail situation (such as ordering in a restaurant or returning a toy to a shop) before trying it with a family member or friend. Remember, genuine assertive communication is based on a real sense of kindness, both to yourself and to the other person. It is about respecting their needs and your own.

☆ Try out some of the responses to advice or criticism. How does it feel to respond candidly or with gentle humour, knowing that you don't need to justify yourself? Experiment until you find responses that feel natural to you. Remember, you are the mum.

13

Changes in your romantic relationship

Becoming a parent is often a transformation that is shared. If you are in a romantic relationship then you will be making the voyage with your partner, and there will be challenges not just for you as an individual but for you both, as a couple. Just as your continued wellbeing is important for your baby, your partner's continued wellbeing and the wellbeing of your relationship are also important for the baby's long-term happiness. The purpose of this chapter is to consider how best to share your adventure with your partner and how to continue to build a strong and supportive relationship with your partner, not just for your own happiness, but also for the benefit of your baby.

TWO JOURNEYS, TAKEN TOGETHER

If you are in a relationship then you are sharing the experience of becoming a parent with your partner. Although you are becoming parents together and falling in love with the same baby, you are, in fact, sharing with each other your experience of your two individual journeys. Differences in your own families of origin, differences in your values, differences in your previous experiences with pregnancy and babies, and differences in your readiness to have a baby create two different experiences. And of course there are differences between being pregnant and supporting a pregnant partner, between giving birth and being a support person at birth, and between breastfeeding and supporting breastfeeding.

In short, becoming Mum is different to becoming Dad. This may sound really obvious, but what you may not appreciate at first is that these differences can mean that your journeys unfold at a different pace and cover different terrain. For example, it is not uncommon for a woman to find that she begins to think of her pregnancy as a special and unique baby and to fall in love with that unique individual before—sometimes months before—her partner does. A woman may even find that she spends her first pregnancy as a 'single mum', even though her partner is completely supportive and excited about becoming a father. She may have this 'single mum' experience because she may start thinking of herself as a mum, and of the pregnancy as a unique and individual baby, from early in the pregnancy, while her partner may not become a dad in his own mind until the birth.

These differences in experiences between yourself and your partner can mean that you have different reactions to events such as miscarriage, preterm birth, childbirth or complications in pregnancy and birth. It is important that you don't expect that you should both react in the same way and that you both respect each other's reactions as healthy and normal. Although you may not respond in the same way, it is still possible to give and receive support, and it is reasonable to expect that your partner will support you in your reaction to these events even if his experience is different. At times, you may find that it is also important to seek support from other women who may have direct understanding of your experiences. In fact, you may well find that other women have a greater understanding of your feelings even if they haven't experienced that particular event themselves.

There are also differences between being a primary caregiver and being a secondary caregiver. Usually, even if both parents are very involved in parenting, there is still a clear primary caregiver during babyhood. It is important to be aware of the differences between being a primary caregiver and being a secondary caregiver so that you can both take these into account and work well together as a team.

A primary caregiver is often:

- ✩ with baby for longer
- ✩ more aware of baby's patterns throughout a 24 hour day (because they are usually with him for a 24 hour day)
- ✩ better at looking after baby and getting things done at the same time
- ✩ taking primary responsibility for night-time parenting
- ✩ taking primary responsibility for interacting with health professionals
- ✩ more likely to miss baby when they are apart
- ✩ more likely to need the other parent to step in when they aren't coping as a parent and to provide back-up with parenting (for example, the other parent may take over night-time parenting while the primary caregiver is sick).

A secondary caregiver is often:

- ✩ with baby for less time
- ✩ working longer hours in paid work
- ✩ more likely to feel stressed or drained due to circumstances outside of family life and may need their partner to provide emotional support for this (for example, for their partner to listen to them talk about a stressful work day)
- ✩ more likely to want an exciting and intense play session with baby, in order to make the most of their time together
- ✩ more likely to need their partner to give them enough space and encouragement to persist in finding their own ways to parent (such as finding their own ways to settle the baby).

Who will be the primary caregiver for your baby? Do you both agree on this? What does this mean for you?

....

....

....

....

....

....

It is important to see how your role as a primary or secondary caregiver may create differences in your parenting so that you are aware that it is your role that is creating these differences, rather than fundamental differences between men and women (women in same-sex relationships or women who are playing the role of secondary caregiver may notice these same differences). Although becoming a mum is different to becoming a dad, as we saw at the beginning of this chapter, there is no need to feel that you have to maintain gender stereotypes in how you parent. There's no reason why a dad can't be a champion at being nurturing, or why a mum can't be fabulous at rough-and-tumble play. As always, be guided by your values.

THE RELATIONSHIP MATTERS TO BABY
In the same way that it is easy to see day-to-day choices as choices between doing something for baby and doing something for yourself, it is easy to see day-to-day choices as choices between doing something for your relationship and doing something for baby. This is equally nonsense. If your romantic relationship is happy and healthy, then this stability supports the emotional health of the two most important people in your baby's life: you and your baby's father or co-parent.

VALUES IN THE RELATIONSHIP
Returning again to the concept of values, let's consider what values you have in relation to your romantic relationship so that you can once again use your unique values as your guide.

What do you value in your romantic relationship? What do you find rewarding in your roles as a wife or partner? What qualities do you hope to show in your romantic relationship?

....

....

....

....

....

....

How do you or did you demonstrate these values before trying to fall pregnant or falling pregnant? How did you and your partner express your love for each other? How did you spend time to together? How did you nourish your relationship?

....

....

....

....

....

Has this changed during your journey to motherhood so far? How do you think it will continue to change?

....

....

....

....

....

....

BUILDING A POSITIVE RELATIONSHIP

Just like when you are building positive relationships with others
in general, in order to build a positive relationship with your
partner you need to be realistic. The first way to be realistic is to
understand that you cannot control your partner's behaviour.
The second is to accept that your partner is who they are. This
doesn't mean that you have to like everything that they do or
think that they are right. No doubt your partner has his fair share
of faults and is often wrong! It just means accepting that their
personality, characteristics and faults are what they are. When
this is accepted you can then figure out the best way for you to
act in order to build a better relationship and get your needs met.

IGNORE THE BAD, REWARD THE GOOD

The same principle that we saw in Chapter 12 also applies here.
While you cannot control the behaviour of your partner, the
most effective way to encourage him to do more of what you'd
like him to do is to reward him for these behaviours. Once again,
however, although this approach does work, our instinct is
usually to do the opposite. We tend to complain when he isn't
doing what we want him to do and take it for granted when he
does something we do want him to do, or we may even criticise him because what he is doing isn't quite right.

For example, let's imagine that a woman wants her husband to improve his settling skills. They've fallen into a pattern
where she is the one who settles the baby, but she would like
her husband to be able to settle the baby too, both because this
will take the pressure off her and also because she feels that
this will help to build a stronger bond between her husband
and their baby. She also feels frustrated about this situation
and is, frankly, angry at her husband that he hasn't persisted
in learning to settle their baby.

The next time her husband is playing with their baby and
the baby starts to become grizzly, her husband starts trying
to calm the baby. However, the baby keeps grizzling, and the
husband begins to look over to his wife instead.

The woman feels her frustration at her husband begin to bubble up. What can she do at this point? If she takes the baby from her husband straight away then she'll deprive him of an opportunity to learn how to settle their baby. If she vents her anger at her husband or criticises his poor settling attempt then she'll make it less likely that he'll try to settle the baby again.

If the woman wants to make it more likely that her husband will persist in settling then she needs to give him encouragement at this point by telling him he's doing a good job of settling their baby (even if it isn't that great!) and perhaps, gently and non-critically, sharing some settling ideas. It is worth noting that this isn't at all about who is right. This woman may be very angry with her husband and believe that he has been lazy in not learning to settle their baby, and she may be right. But what does she want to achieve? Does she want to vent her anger or does she want to increase the chances that her husband will learn how to settle their baby? The bottom line is that she needs to encourage any step that her husband takes towards being able to settle their baby if she wants to increase the chances that he will persist in his attempts, both now and in the future.

CONTINUING TO NOURISH YOUR RELATIONSHIP

Pregnancy and caring for a new baby are likely to create changes in your life that affect the ways in which you and your partner can be together. Even if you begin this journey with an extremely happy relationship, it is easy for this transition to mean that you stop nourishing your relationship. Instead, it is important to make this transition about finding new ways to be together and new ways to support each other that fit with your new life. Use your values as a basis for finding new joint activities and new ways to nourish your relationship. Just like with building a rewarding life, it is important that you think small. Often we can easily think of the big ways to nourish our romantic relationship, such as a date night. If you have time for a date night every so often that is fantastic, but a date takes a lot of effort and organisation, especially with a baby. It is important therefore to remember to nourish our relationship regularly with smaller acts; for example, asking, 'How was your day?' and listening to the reply. When you have a baby, this is a much easier way to maintain your relationship than going on a date!

It is also important to continue nourishing your relationship regardless of any current disputes or arguments. In other words, don't withdraw from nourishing your relationship in order to punish your partner. Although it is tempting at times, this simply won't help you to improve your relationship; on the contrary, it will only make things worse. In fact, actually increasing your efforts to nourish your relationship, while at the same time assertively communicating your desires in the area of the dispute, is much more likely to lead to a resolution in your favour.

List ways that you can continue to support each other based on your values and the ways that you like to nourish your relationship. Remember to think small:

....

....

....

....

....

....

Here are some ideas for small acts that you can both do to nourish your relationship:

- ☆ Ask 'how was your day?' and listen to the reply.
- ☆ Say 'I love you'.
- ☆ Praise each other's parenting.
- ☆ Say 'thank you'.
- ☆ Make each other hot drinks, meals or snacks.

- ✫ Give each other hugs and cuddles.
- ✫ Share a kiss or two.
- ✫ Take a walk together (wearing your baby in a sling/possum pouch, or with baby in a pram).
- ✫ Play with baby together.
- ✫ Compliment each other.
- ✫ Talk about shared interests and daily activities (remembering to talk not just about the baby, but also about working life, wider family, friends and joint interests).
- ✫ Watch a movie or show together (maybe cuddling or feeding baby at the same time).
- ✫ Offer back-up for one another when a break is needed.

SEX AND NOURISHING YOUR RELATIONSHIP

Sex is an important aspect of a relationship, and for many couples an active sex life plays a key role in nourishing their relationship. It is normal to experience changes to your sex life due to the pressure of trying to conceive, the symptoms of pregnancy, the effects of hormonal changes on your sex drive, the time required to heal after birth, fatigue, and the realities of caring for a newborn baby. In a long-term sexual relationship a continued, mutually enjoyable sex life requires open and honest communication, good understanding of your (and your partner's) unique sexuality, flexibility, and an optimistic outlook that turns temporary obstacles into sexual opportunities.

If sex plays a central role in nourishing your relationship, this may be an opportunity to future-proof your relationship so that sex remains satisfying for years to come. Communicate with each other about your unique sexualities and values in relation to physical intimacy. What is important about sex to you?

Be prepared to be flexible. Sex becomes a habit like any other, and it is likely that before trying to fall pregnant, you and your partner fell into a rhythm that worked for you both at the time. The changes brought from conception, pregnancy and birth are likely to disrupt that rhythm, but you can find a new rhythm to suit your new circumstances. It is easy to fall into the trap of reducing good sex into an equation like an exact frequency or a particular sexual act. In fact, there are many and varied ways to have a sex life that is mutually satisfying.

Finally, have an optimistic outlook. Temporary setbacks to your sex life may be opportunities to experiment with new ways to be sexual and to reinvigorate your sex life in the long-term. It is also important not to make sex conditional. Remember that withdrawing nourishment from the relationship as a punishment is likely to make things worse, whereas increasing your efforts to nourish the relationship while also assertively maintaining your position in the argument is more likely to achieve a satisfactory resolution.

PARENTING TOGETHER

Becoming an effective and happy parenting team requires open and honest communication and mutual respect. It is important to have open, clear communication about your parenting values. Remember, when we have a good sense of the values that underlie our decisions, it is then easier to be flexible and to adapt our actions to specific circumstances in a way that still fits with our values. In the same way, by having a good sense of not just your values in relation to parenting but also your partner's values, it is easier for you to figure out the best way to parent together and how to compromise best in areas where you disagree.

Initiate lots of discussion about parenting values. You can initiate a discussion by explaining the concept of values and talking about your own values as a mum. It is also useful to clarify the values that underlie your partner's opinions on specific parenting issues. When you are discussing values with your partner, do remember that you are both taking different journeys at a different pace. For example, while you may have a clear sense of your values as a mum during pregnancy, your partner may not yet have a clear sense of his values as a dad until after the baby is born. Also remember that assertive communication is about communicating with acceptance of both yourself and of your partner, and with respect for both of your needs.

There will be times when you disagree. In resolving disputes over parenting you may find it helpful to try some of the following suggestions:

- ✰ Bring the dispute to the level of values. Instead of arguing about the specifics, clarify the values that are underlying each of your desires. Is it possible for you to live out both of these values by taking a different approach? Or is it possible for one of you to compromise your values in this specific area if you ensure that this value is lived out in other ways?

- ✰ Sidestep debates about what is the best thing to do and instead stick to assertively expressing how you feel. Instead of getting caught in a debate about what's right, make the discussion about figuring out how to parent together in a way that will keep you both happy.

- ✰ Sometimes you'll find that you have the same values but disagree on how they are best lived. Is this an issue where seeking professional advice, getting further information on infant development or talking to other parents may help?

- ✰ Sometimes you can take different approaches. For example, if one of you strongly values encouraging musical development and the other does not, that parent alone can encourage musical development.

- ✰ Are you stuck in an either/or argument, debating between two alternatives? If so, it may help to brainstorm and get ideas from other parents so that you've considered all possible alternatives. There may be a third option that is satisfactory to both of you.

- ✰ Are you able to agree on what a good outcome is? If you can agree on what an effective approach would look like in practice, then you can agree to try different ideas and stick with what works.

WHAT IF MY PARTNER JUST ISN'T PLAYING THE GAME?

Remember that you cannot change your partner's behaviour, only your own. A happy, healthy romantic relationship requires input from both parties. Often, when we change our behaviour towards our partner by remembering to do things that nourish our relationship (such as giving him a hug and a kiss when you are reunited after a day apart), when we communicate our needs assertively and when we reward our partner with thank-yous and compliments when he does what we want him to do, then his behaviour will change and our relationship will became happier. However, if you are making an effort to do all of these things and your relationship still isn't getting any better, then maybe your partner simply isn't willing to change.

The question for you then is, if your partner isn't willing to change, if your relationship isn't going to get any easier or happier, is it worth staying? Of course, any partner is going to have faults that won't change and that you'll need to learn to live with. We cannot expect perfection. It is also true, though, that some people have faults that are incompatible with having a healthy, happy romantic relationship. Learning to live with a partner who is chronically messy is one thing; learning to live with a partner who is chronically selfish is another thing entirely. If your romantic relationship is happy and healthy (or can become so), it is valuable to your baby as it can provide stability to you all. However, if it isn't happy and healthy then it doesn't provide that stability, and baby's interests may be better served by relying on other support people and making yourself available for a happy and healthy relationship with someone else. Sometimes the best outcome, even if you still love your partner, is for the relationship to end.

If you are unsure about whether to leave or stay, try talking it through with a support person whom you trust. Consider whether you are able to be the mum that you want to be within this relationship. Are you able to live your values in other areas of your life (values in relation to career, family, and friends) within this relationship? Are you able to be the kind of romantic partner that you want to be within this relationship? Is your partner abusive? Emotional abuse may include your partner controlling your life; for example, limiting your access to money, controlling how you dress or controlling who you see. Emotional abuse can also include frequent criticism and ridicule as well as using verbal threats and intimidation. Unfortunately, sometimes emotional or physical abuse can begin during pregnancy right when you are most vulnerable and most in need of your partner's support. If this has been your experience, know that you are not alone and it is not your fault. Your greatest strengths (kindness, forgiveness, an easygoing attitude) may be exactly what made you blind to the warning signs. It is vital in evaluating your relationship to also consider the needs of your baby. In becoming a mum your relationship decisions are no longer entirely about your own happiness. You must therefore also consider whether you are able to keep your baby safe from experiencing emotional or physical abuse from your partner. What kind of father are you giving your baby if you stay?

If you are experiencing significant relationship difficulties and you feel that the relationship may be salvageable, you may consider seeking professional help, and assertively communicating your desire for such help to your partner. The alternative to seeking help, or the option you may come to if the professional help doesn't work, is to leave. Sometimes, even when two people love each other, the best resolution for one or both of the individuals in the relationship is still for the relationship to end.

Ending a relationship means going through the pain of a broken heart. It may also mean confronting fears of being unable to find another romantic partner as well as the challenges of single motherhood. If you are contemplating ending your relationship, then you have my full sympathy for the pain and the difficulty of your situation. With that fully acknowledged, it is important to consider this: do you want to make your life about avoiding the pain of a broken heart or about being the best mum you can be? This is not an easy question and you may feel yourself trying to recoil from it. Stay with the question. Connect with your values as a mum and imagine your child, all grown up, talking about you as a mum; what do you hope for her to say? For example, if your partner is abusive, imagine your child saying proudly, 'The thing I love about my mum is she always kept me safe, even when that meant experiencing a broken heart . . . '. Stop and really imagine it. Does that resonate? Connect to your values in other areas of your life. Will leaving your relationship, though painful, allow you to be the person you want to be?

ONE WOMAN'S STORY
Reading Megan's story may help you to build a stronger relationship with your own partner.
When Megan and Christopher decided to start trying to fall pregnant, it was very much a joint decision and they both felt equally ready to become parents. So when Megan fell pregnant after only three months of trying they were both equally thrilled. Megan was surprised then at how differently they experienced the pregnancy. She felt like she became a mum the moment that she found out that she was pregnant. Early on, she found herself with responsibilities to protect and nurture her baby. She had to avoid alcohol and specific foods, get regular gentle exercise and get a good night's sleep. She also found herself quickly called upon to make sacrifices for her baby—like her breakfast every morning! In contrast, Chris's life, however, continued as normal.

When Megan experienced a miscarriage at nine weeks she felt utterly devastated. Chris was also disappointed, but it was different. Chris was disappointed that their plans to have a child were now delayed. In contrast, Megan grieved for that particular baby. When Megan fell pregnant again several months later, she again fell in love with that specific baby from the beginning. Megan and Chris were both anxious about another miscarriage, but for Megan alone this meant a moment of heart-thumping fear every time she went to the bathroom and a moment of relief when she saw that there was no blood on her underwear.

Megan and Chris both became increasingly relieved and excited as her pregnancy continued to progress. Although they each experienced their own journey in becoming a parent, they were able to support each other in their own reactions and experiences. Megan felt that it was vital for her to use assertive communication with Chris, stating her needs openly and honestly in a way that was respectful to him. For example, Megan was clear in communicating to Chris that she needed him to attend antenatal classes with her and to discuss her birth plan with her, so that she could be confident that he would be able to support her fully as a birth partner. She also found that she needed to be assertive in communicating her desires for the nursery, as Chris reacted to her pregnancy by becoming increasingly concerned about their finances. For example, Megan was clear in communicating that it was important to her to have a comfortable rocking chair for settling baby and for feeding. With assertive communication it was clear that Megan's desire for a rocking chair was driven by her values regarding physical affection and breastfeeding, whereas Chris' reluctance to buy the chair came from his own values regarding providing financially for the family in the long-term. Once they were clear that they didn't disagree on their values, and with insight into how their different anticipated roles as primary and secondary caregivers were colouring their own perspectives, Megan and Chris then were able to problem-solve how they would ensure that Megan had all the equipment she wanted for the nursery while keeping an eye on their finances at the same time.

After baby Isabelle was born Megan knew that she needed to give Chris sufficient space to find his footing as the dad. She was conscious of supporting him in his parenting, and when he took on a task that she normally performed (as the primary caregiver), she let him do it his way. She was also conscious of being encouraging whenever Chris took a step in the right direction. Over time they found that they developed different ways of settling Isabelle, with Megan using the rocking chair and singing lullabies and Chris taking the baby for a walk in the pram.

Megan and Chris also found that with baby Isabelle in their lives they needed to change the ways that they spent time together as a couple. They decided to make a conscious effort always to ask each other how their day was and to listen to the reply. They were also conscious of the little ways that they could brighten each other's day and continue to nurture their relationship, such as making each other a cup of tea or coffee, or sharing a cuddle. Most days it took a lot of effort to settle Isabelle to sleep, and Chris and Megan developed an evening routine of taking the baby for a walk in her pram to help her settle to sleep. As they walked, and Isabelle slowly settled to sleep, Chris and Megan were able to connect, chatting to each other, holding each other's hands and sharing a kiss or two.

MY UNIQUE ADVENTURE
These comments may help you to understand how the information in this chapter might relate to your unique experience.

Help! This wasn't what I had planned!
May be relevant to women experiencing difficulty conceiving, miscarriage, complications, preterm birth, an unwanted birth experience or finding motherhood different from expectations.
The unexpected challenges of pregnancy, birth and parenthood can be experienced very differently between yourself and your partner. Although you are in a sense sharing your journey to parenthood with your partner, in many ways you are on two different journeys. It is important to remember that it is healthy and normal for you to have different reactions to some challenges. Despite this, it is still reasonable to expect to support each other. Ensure that you support your partner in his reaction even if it is different from your own, and use assertive communication to communicate your experiences and make clear the ways that he can support you. It may be important also to

connect with other women for emotional support, particularly those who have experienced similar challenges.

Grief and loss

May be relevant to any woman experiencing a loss, whether it be an obvious loss such as miscarriage or stillbirth, or the loss of pre-motherhood life, difficulty conceiving, an unwanted birth experience or motherhood being different from expectations.

Just as there are differences between being pregnant and being the partner of a pregnant woman, and between giving birth and being a support person for a birth, you may find that if you experience a loss that your partner experiences the loss very differently. It is important, first of all, to acknowledge that it is healthy and natural for you to have different reactions to loss and to grieve in different ways. It is also reasonable to expect your partner to be supportive of you in your grief even if he isn't experiencing a similar grief reaction. It is important to use assertive communication to make clear to your partner how you are feeling, your needs and how you'd like him to support you. You may feel that it is also important to turn to other women, particularly women who have experienced a similar loss, for understanding emotional support.

Two Mummies

May be relevant to women in same-sex relationships.

If you are in a same-sex relationship you will still find that you are sharing two different journeys. Your partner and you may still have differences in families of origin, values, previous experiences with pregnancy and babies, and differences in your readiness to have a baby. If pregnancy, childbirth, breastfeeding and being the primary caregiver is going to be the domain of one of you alone, you may find that this creates additional differences in your journeys just as it does for heterosexual couples. It is important to recognise that this is normal. Healthy, happy same-sex partnerships are made with the same ingredients as healthy, happy heterosexual partnerships: communicate well, reward your partner when they take a step in the right direction and nourish your relationship. How you parent should be based on your unique values, not on gender stereotypes. There's no reason why you can't both be fantastic mums who, together, meet your baby's needs.

Adoption
May be relevant to mums waiting to adopt or new mums of adopted babies.

If you are adopting a child then you may find that the experience of becoming a parent is more similar for yourself and your partner than it is for natural parents. However, there may still be differences in how you make the transition to parenthood caused by differences in families of origin, values, previous experiences with pregnancy and babies, or different roles as primary or secondary caregivers. Good communication and regularly nourishing your relationship is still key to long-term happiness as a couple.

PUTTING IT INTO PRACTICE

✮ Discuss with your partner the ways that you think your relationship may change with baby. Talk about how you currently nurture your relationship and what is important to both of you in terms of how you spend time together and express your love for each other. Then think about how you can continue to nurture your relationship once your baby arrives. Remember to think of plenty of small actions that you can take.

✮ Make an effort to do more of the small actions that nurture your relationship. Does this make a difference? Do you find yourself more connected to your partner?

✮ Notice how you respond when your partner does something that you want him to do. Are you good at ignoring the bad and rewarding the good? Make sure that when he does something you want him to do, you reward this by saying thank you. If he has taken longer than you wanted, or he isn't doing it quite right, bite your tongue for now! Remember that you need to encourage this first step if you want him to take another.

☆ Remember that although you are becoming parents together, you are taking two different journeys. You may find that there are times when your partner doesn't understand your current experiences on the path to parenthood (and vice versa). You may find it important to talk to other women, particularly women who have been in similar circumstances. Although you are going to experience the journey differently, you can still fully support each other in your own unique experiences.

☆ Practise assertive communication with your partner. Remember that this is based on a respect for both his needs and your own. Communicate your own needs as directly and openly as you can. Assertive communication takes practice, so keep practising.

14

Returning
to values

Just as all babies are unique, every woman's journey to mother-hood is unique, with different women experiencing different challenges. This book is all about helping you to become the mum that you want to be. This means finding your unique values as a mum and basing your decisions and behaviour day to day on these values rather than on avoiding pain, on worry-ing thoughts or on what other people say. In this chapter we return to your mothering values and begin to explore, in a more concrete way, how you are going to mother based on these values. This includes exploring the implications of your values for specific experiences such as birth, as well as setting goals that you can begin acting on today.

YOUR UNIQUE MOTHERING VALUES
At the beginning of this book I asked you to explore your unique mothering values. Before we begin to think about how, in a more concrete way, you are going to live out your mothering values, let's redo the exercises that you completed at the begin-ning of the book.

Imagine being able, unseen and unheard, to watch and hear your child (or your future child if you are trying to conceive) as an adult, 20 or 30 years in the future. In your mind's eye allow yourself to imagine your child, all grown up, going about her daily life. What do you wish for her? What do you hope her to be like? What characteristics do you hope to have fostered in her? See your child interacting with workmates and friends; imagine her in love, imagine her interacting with her own children.

I want to encourage my child to grow into an adult who is:

....

....

....

....

....

Imagine that your child shows those exact characteristics that you are hoping to encourage. Consider what actions you may have taken as a mother to have encouraged these characteristics in your child.

As a mother, I may have contributed to the development of my child's characteristics by:

....

....

....

....

....

Now imagine that you are watching your child, as an adult, reflect on her own childhood. Perhaps you might like to imagine that she is talking about her childhood with a partner or with a friend. What memories of her childhood do you hope to hear her recall? Imagine that she begins to discuss you, as a mother. What would you hope to hear her say about you? You probably would love to hear her say that you were a good mother, but try to push past that to the specifics. Imagine her completing one of the following sentences: 'The thing that's really special about my mum is . . . ' or 'I'll always be grateful to my mum for . . . ' or 'I'm lucky I had the mum I had because . . . '.

As a mother, the impression I want to leave on my child is:

....

....

....

....

....

Now imagine that you are transported from Earth to a special, magical place with your child. In this special place it is just you and your child as a newborn baby. If you are currently trying to conceive or are pregnant, imagine that in this magical place you are with your baby as a newborn. There is no one else here to judge you and no pressure to achieve anything in particular as a mother. Your baby is alert and calm. Your baby is just happy to be with you and doesn't need anything in particular right now. Somehow you just know that in this special, magical place you can do whatever you want as a mother with the guarantee that no harm will come to your baby. You are both completely protected, so there is no pressure to get anything right. This is just a special time for you to *enjoy* your baby. If you could simply *enjoy* being a mum without the need to do anything 'right', without fear of judgment from others, without pressure from the outside world or from baby's needs, what would you do?

As a mother, I enjoy my baby by:

....

....

....

....

....

....

GREATER CLARITY

Compare your answers now to your answers at the beginning
of the book. Are there any changes? Have some of your values
as a mum become clearer to you? How might qualities such as
mindfulness, acceptance or kindness fit with becoming the
mum that you want to be?

....

....

....

....

....

Look at the qualities that you want your baby to show as an
adult and consider, again, how you could encourage those characteristics in light of everything you have learned in reading
this book. Some of the links between your mothering and the
characteristics your child may have as an adult are easy to see.
For example, it is probably clear to you that if you want your
child to grow into an adult who is physically affectionate then
it is important to show him lots of physical affection. However,
you may also find characteristics that you want to encourage
in your child but you aren't sure how to do it.

You may also find that you have intuitive theories on how
to encourage particular characteristics in your baby that may
not, in fact, be correct. Reconsider the ways in which you can
encourage particular characteristics using everything that you
have learned in this book. For example, you may wish for your
child to grow into an adult who leads a happy and fulfilled life.

It might seem like the best way to encourage this is to stop your baby from experiencing any negative feelings. You now know, however, that the pain and the joys in life are attached and that trying to avoid pain is not, ultimately, the best way to a happy and fulfilled life. As a mum, you can create the bedrock of future happiness by reacting to your baby's emotions, painful or not, with acceptance and love, thus encouraging your baby to be accepting of his own emotions. Similarly, you may value your child growing into an adult who is independent and confident. It may seem like the best way to encourage this is to ensure that your baby is independent in sleeping, soothing or feeding from the beginning by firmly ignoring any cries and giving your baby plenty of time alone to fend for himself. In fact, however, it is the love and responsiveness that you provide now that gives your baby the foundation of security and acceptance on which adult independence and confidence can later be built.

Returning to our summary of baby's needs in Chapter 9, 'Loving baby', the greatest gifts that you can give your baby is to accept him for who he is in the here and now, to notice what he needs and, as best you can, to respond to these needs. It may also be the case that you need more information on infant development or on how you can encourage your baby to develop the characteristics that you wish for him as an adult. We'll look at infant development now.

UNDERSTANDING YOUR NEWBORN BABY

To help you understand your newborn baby better and hence to understand how you can best live out your values as a new mum, here are some quick facts about infant development.

- ✫ Human newborns are more like foetuses than babies (just think about a human newborn in comparison to a newborn horse that can walk around the paddock hours after birth). It is therefore normal for a human baby to be highly dependent on her parents and to have a high need for physical closeness.
- ✫ Lots of love and acceptance during babyhood and lots of mum responding to baby's cues creates the foundation of

acceptance and security on which adult confidence, independence and self-soothing can all later be built.

✩ It isn't possible to spoil a baby. Babyhood is all about baby learning new skills and behaviours, and about baby learning that what he does makes a difference. As a baby grows, more and more of his behaviour is learned (learned, *not* manipulative). For example, an older baby might call out 'Ga! Ga!' when he is hungry, and his mum might respond by offering the breast or a bottle. This older baby has learned to call out in order to get milk. It might seem strange, but this kind of learning is actually the bedrock for good behaviour later on. With time, 'Ga! Ga!' turns into 'Mum!', then, 'Mum, I'm hungry', and eventually, 'Excuse me, Mum. I'm going to make a sandwich. Would you like one?' During babyhood, the important point is that baby is learning that there are things that he can do to control his world and get his needs met. As he grows up you can expect his behaviours to become more sophisticated.

✩ It is normal for babies to experience intense emotional reactions, and it is normal in these situations for a baby to seek comfort from mum (or another adult). It is also normal for there to be times when it is difficult to calm your baby and other times when she calms really quickly. When she calms very quickly, this may seem strange to you and you might wonder if she was manipulating you. Although babies do learn that crying brings attention, they are not capable of manipulating adults (for example, a baby can't think, 'I know I'll pretend to be upset by crying and then mum will think that I'm upset and she'll come running'). They just don't have the language or the ability to imagine the mental states of others that is required for true manipulation. A baby's emotions can fluctuate so quickly (for better and for worse) because babies don't have the ability to moderate their emotions with language. This means that they can't give themselves calming self-talk when something goes wrong for them, and it also means that they can't dwell on situations either.

☆ It is normal for babies to wake during the night and to need help to settle to sleep. This does improve naturally with time, but even at one year of age waking up during the night is so common that it really can't be considered abnormal. As with all developmental milestones (such as rolling over or crawling), there is real variability in when babies learn to soothe themselves to sleep and when they learn to sleep through the night.

Do these facts about infant development change any of your ideas about how you can, as a mum, best support your baby growing up into the adult you'd like your baby to be? Do you need to get more information on infant development?

If you have questions about infant development, write them down here for future reference.

....

....

....

....

....

....

If you are intending to breastfeed, don't forget to also get information on breastfeeding. Unfortunately, it is still common for women to receive incorrect advice on breastfeeding, including from health professionals. If you are intending to breastfeed, it is vital to ensure that you are accessing the right advice when you need it. It is ideal to be armed with an accurate understanding of breastfeeding during pregnancy. Make sure that this includes not just information on how to breastfeed but also information on your options if you experience challenges with breastfeeding. These options may include exclusive expressing (expressing breast milk and feeding it to baby from a bottle), using a supplementary nursing system (delivering complementary expressed breast milk or formula to baby from a tube connected to your breast, so that baby is still suckling at your breast regularly in order to increase your milk supply and to learn how to get milk directly from the breast), deliberately increasing milk supply (such as by giving baby frequent long feeds or expressing frequently, or with herbal supplements or medication if you have been given medical advice that this may be beneficial for you) and using a nipple shield for your own comfort if your baby's suckling is painful.

There are two avenues to receiving accurate breastfeeding information. The first is from mother-led breastfeeding support organisations such as La Leche League International (http://www.llli.org) and the Australian Breastfeeding Association (https://www.breastfeeding.asn.au). Both organisations have excellent resources online, and the Australian Breastfeeding Association has a free counselling service for Australian mums.

The second is seeking professional advice from a qualified lactation consultant. A qualified lactation consultant is a health professional with specialist knowledge on breastfeeding. Other health professionals may not have specialist knowledge on breastfeeding and may give advice that is not consistent with the latest research.

Do you need to get more information on breastfeeding? If so, write any questions that you have here for future reference.

....

....

....

....

....

....

How would you summarise your values as a mum now?

....

....

....

....

....

....

Look through your summary of your mothering values one last time. Are there any values that are clearly more important to you than others?

If you could live by only one of the values that you have written down, which would you choose? Do you have one (or two) key values?

....

....

....

....

....

It is important to understand what your key values are because there may be times when you'll need to prioritise.

THE IMPLICATIONS OF MY VALUES

Now that you have greater clarity about what your values are, are there implications of your values for trying to fall pregnant, pregnancy, birth and life as a new mum? In considering this, don't merely consider how you'd like to live out your values if everything goes according to plan. Remember that there are many aspects of this journey that you cannot control, from how long it takes you to fall pregnant, to how the pregnancy unfolds, to how the birth proceeds, to what exactly your baby is like. Think about how you can best live out your values in the best- and the worst-case scenarios, as well as everything in between.

Do your values have implications for trying to fall pregnant; for example, your lifestyle while you are trying to fall? Are there things that you want to learn to do before you fall pregnant? How will you live out your values if you have difficulty falling pregnant? Would you consider IVF or adoption? If so, how will you approach these options?

....

....

....

....

....

....

....

Do your values have implications for pregnancy; for example, are there implications for your lifestyle while you are pregnant? Are there goals you'd like to set for yourself during your pregnancy? Are there things that you'd like to achieve to prepare yourself for baby's arrival? Are there implications for how you will handle the symptoms of pregnancy such as morning sickness? Are there implications for how you'll handle any complications that arise?

....

....

....

....

....

....

....

Do your values have implications for birth? Is there a particular way in which you'd like to give birth? Do your values have implications in terms of pain relief, interventions or support people in birth? Which aspects of your birth plan are high priority and which are low priority? Remember to consider how you would live out your values in birth if the birth doesn't go according to plan (such as if you had to have an emergency caesarean, or needed pain relief that you would ideally prefer to not have).

....

....

....

....

....

....

....

Do your values have implications for your life as a new mum? Are there implications for your lifestyle? Are there goals that you'd like to set for yourself in your time as a new mum? Again, remember to consider how you would live out your values if things don't go according to plan (for example, if your baby needs to spend time in hospital after birth).

....

....

....

....

....

....

....

Do your values have implications for how you want to handle sleeping, feeding or settling? For example, is it important to you to co-sleep or to sleep separately; to breastfeed, to bottle feed formula or to bottle feed expressed breast milk? Are there particular ways of settling that you favour? You may not have strong preferences based on your values, and that is okay. However, if you do have preferences based on your values, consider exactly why you have each preference—that is, what value it relates to. Also consider what you will prioritise, based on your values. For example, if your values strongly support breastfeeding and you don't have strong values regarding sleeping, then it makes sense always to handle sleeping in a way that promotes breastfeeding, such as breastfeeding baby to sleep when that suits you and your baby. What are any implications of your values for how you want to handle sleeping, feeding or settling?

....

....

....

....

....

....

Remember that things may well not go according to plan. For example, if you would prefer to breastfeed but you have difficulty breastfeeding, would you consider using nipple shields or expressing breast milk and feeding it to baby from a bottle? And how will you continue to live out your values if you have to bottle feed formula? How will you continue to live out your values if things don't turn out as you'd prefer?

....

....

....

....

....

....

Look through these implications. There may be some areas in which you have strong preferences based on your values and other areas in which you don't have any real preference. Remember that your own energy is limited and, as mums, we can't do everything.

What are your priorities?

....

....

....

....

....

....

Further, it is vital that you remember that there are many aspects of the journey that you cannot control. Even if you have a strong preference for your pregnancy, birth or early mothering experience to be a certain way, based on your values, this may not happen, but you can still find ways to live your values. For example, many women may have strong preferences for their birth experience. A particular woman may realise that, all other things being equal, she'd love to have a drug-free vaginal birth. It is good to know what your own preferences are, but it isn't good to become inflexible about them. The reality is that we cannot control perfectly whether or not we have a drug-free vaginal birth. Thus, this woman has to consider how she can still live out her values as best she can if she has to have an emergency caesarean. This is about being flexible. If we keep ourselves connected to our values, rather than just to our plans or our goals, we can be flexible. We can ask ourselves if our plans or our goals are working in the situations that we find ourselves in and with our unique baby. And if they aren't working then we can adapt them, based on our values.

GOALS FOR NOW

Now consider where you currently are in your journey. Are there any goals that you'd like to set yourself for the upcoming months? Remember that a goal is something that you can achieve and tick off your list. It is important when making goals to ensure that they are achievable and realistic. It is easy to think of big goals, but try to bring your thinking down to size and set yourself goals that are small. For example, if you'd like to take regular walks during pregnancy, don't make the goal huge like walking for an hour every day. Make it smaller and more realistic, like walking for 20 minutes, three to four times a week. By realistic, I mean something that you know you'll be able to do. Remember, it is always possible to exceed your goal and take an extra walk!

My goals for the upcoming months:

....

....

....

....

....

....

....

Looking over your goals, are there any barriers to you achieving them? If so, what are they?

....

....

....

....

....

....

If there are barriers, can you remove the barrier by making the goal smaller? Sometimes we see a barrier because the goal we've set simply isn't realistic. If this isn't the case, is the barrier really one of your monsters talking? Is the barrier a thought or an emotion? If so, think about how you can use the skills in previous chapters of this book to overcome this.

If the barrier isn't a monster, you may need to do some practical problem-solving. Take some time to work out how to remove any barriers that may prevent you from achieving your goal.

Is there someone in your support network who could help you to overcome the barrier? Would discussing this barrier with your midwife, doctor or child health nurse help? Would doing some research online or from books help you to come up with ideas?

....

....

....

....

....

....

The next step is to begin to work towards your goals. This will be dealt with in more detail in the next chapter.

ONE WOMAN'S STORY

Reading Jennifer's story may help you to be flexible and to live out your values in the circumstances in which you find yourself. Jennifer found that she and her husband Ahmed had to revise their plans for feeding and sleeping when their baby girl Emily was born. Before Emily's birth Jennifer and Ahmed had set up her cot in the nursery, and they were planning for Emily to sleep in this from day one, even for her daytime naps. Jennifer was also determined to breastfeed. When Emily was born, however, they found that she just would not stay asleep once they put her into the cot. It seemed that their baby would stay sleep only as long as she was in someone's arms. Jennifer and Ahmed spent their first week of parenthood taking turns staying up at night holding a sleeping baby Emily.

Jennifer also had much more difficulty breastfeeding than she had anticipated. It was difficult getting baby Emily to latch on properly, and Jennifer's nipples were quickly munched into sore, bleeding, cracked lumps of flesh. Every feed was excruciatingly painful. It felt like having razor blades drawn over her flesh. Jennifer spent her first week as a mum dreading feeding times, and Ahmed often found her weeping after feeds in pain and frustration. They both knew that they had to revise their plans.

Jennifer and Ahmed started by going back to their values. They thought through the values underpinning their plans to have baby Emily sleep in her nursery and to breastfeed. Their values underlying their decision to put Emily to sleep in a cot in the nursery were wishing to keep Emily safe and thinking that having Emily sleep in a cot in the nursery would enable them have time to pursue their own values as individuals, as well as to have time together as a couple in order to keep their marriage strong. Their values underlying the desire to breastfeed were valuing baby Emily's physical health in the long term and wanting to promote bonding through feeding. However, things certainly weren't going according to plan, as Jennifer and Ahmed weren't getting any time to themselves at all and, far from being a pleasant bonding experience, Jennifer was finding the pain of breastfeeding an obstacle to bonding with Emily and enjoying motherhood.

Once they were clear on their values, the couple then sought professional advice from their local maternity and child health nurse and from a lactation consultant. They were advised that moving baby Emily's cot into their bedroom would actually be safer for the baby and could help her to stay sleep (as she'd be able to hear Jennifer and Ahmed). The maternal and child health nurse assured them that it was normal for a newborn baby to have a high need for physical contact and suggested that they try carrying Emily in a possum pouch/sling during the day. Following an assessment, the lactation consultant was confident that baby Emily had tongue tie (the flesh that connects the tongue to the floor of the mouth was shorter than usual, restricting tongue movement) and referred them to a doctor with expertise in tongue tie to confirm diagnosis and consider a simple surgical correction to release the tongue.

Jennifer and Ahmed, guided by their values, decided to move baby Emily's cot into their bedroom that night and were relieved to find that she did sleep more soundly in their room. They also began to wear Emily using a possum pouch during the day, and found that the baby would sleep well in the possum pouch. This meant that Jennifer was free to fulfil her own needs and individual values while still giving baby Emily the physical contact that she needed.

Jennifer also decided that while she was waiting to see the doctor about tongue tie she would express her milk and feed it to baby Emily from a bottle. While she was feeding baby Emily from a bottle she continued to live her value of promoting bonding through feeding by feeding Emily based on Emily's cues and giving her plenty of physical affection at every feed. After the tongue tie was fixed, Jennifer decided to take a gradual approach to returning to breastfeeding. She continued expressing her milk and feeding Emily from a bottle for some feeds. She also used a nipple shield for her first feeds directly from the breast. Jennifer had become fearful of breastfeeding, so taking a gradual approach allowed her to ease back into it. Jennifer experienced some criticism from friends and family but she knew that this decision was right for her. Taking a gradual approach helped Jennifer to focus on bonding with baby Emily, and it was this that mattered most to her.

MY UNIQUE ADVENTURE

These comments may help you to understand how the information in this chapter might relate to your unique experience.

Becoming a confident mum

May be relevant to women at any stage who are struggling to find confidence in their own mothering, coping with self-doubt or coping with criticism and advice from others.

Finding confidence as a mum is about finding how to apply your values to the unique situations in which you find yourself with your unique baby. As you set goals based on your values, adapt your goals to suit what works with your unique baby, and then achieve your goals, you will gradually find yourself becoming more confident in your own judgment.

Help! This wasn't what I had planned!

May be relevant to women experiencing difficulty conceiving, miscarriage, pregnancy complications, preterm birth, an unwanted birth experience or finding motherhood different from expectations.

There are many aspects of the journey to motherhood that we simply cannot control. It is important to think about how we can live out our values when circumstances don't go according to plan. Often this may take some creativity. We can become stuck in the plans that we have created and the goals that we've set. If you find yourself getting stuck in thinking about what you were planning to do, ask yourself why that mattered. What was the value underlying that plan or goal? After reconnecting with your values you can spend some time thinking of ways that you can live out the value now. Remember that you may need to truly think small. If you are having difficulty, you may find it helpful to brainstorm with a support person who knows you well, or with other women in similar circumstances.

PUTTING IT INTO PRACTICE

☆ Make a list of the goals that you can be working on right now and put this somewhere to remind yourself. You can tick off your goals as you achieve them.

☆ Think through how your values apply during pregnancy, while giving birth and as a new mum. Think about whether your values have implications in terms of sleeping, feeding or settling. Remember, don't just think about how your values can be lived in the ideal situation. There are many things that you cannot fully control. How can you best live out your values if everything doesn't go according to plan? What are your priorities?

☆ When planning what you'd like to do regarding giving birth, or with sleeping, feeding and settling as a new mum, be very clear about what values underpin these plans. The clearer you are on what your values are, the more flexible you can be. Remember that while you may have your plan, your baby may have another plan entirely! Adapt your plans in the situation by considering what is *working* for you and for your baby in the context of your values.

15

Acting on mothering values

Being the mum that you want to be is not about who you are or are not when you begin the journey, but what you do along the way. In fact, it is the sum total of a million little somethings done again and again, day by day, on good days and on bad days. It takes a million little acts of love—a cuddle here, a kiss there—to build a loving mum. How do you actually take those steps? How do you start *doing* being the mum you want to be?

This chapter is where we get concrete. In the previous chapter you created goals for how you could start being the mum that you want to be in a way that is relevant for you now. In this chapter we explore actually acting on your goals and incorporating small acts into your day.

AND HERE COME THE MONSTERS

A sure way to get your monsters to come out to play is to begin to do things that you value. As you start moving in the right direction you may find that your monsters become very ugly and very loud. So, a woman with the *I must be a perfect mum* monster who decides to start reading to her baby will hear a lot of chatter about how she must read a book every day and how she must read it perfectly. A woman with the *I'm not a good enough mum* monster who decides to take her baby to a mother's group will hear a lot of chatter about how she isn't as good as all the other mums. A woman with the *It shouldn't be like this* monster who is enjoying cuddling her sleeping baby will hear chatter about how her baby should be sleeping in his cot.

Why is that? Well, it is to do with what we explored fully in Chapter 2: our pain and our joys are attached. Moving in the right direction then will probably involve moving towards, not away from, our pain. When you start to move in the right direction you'll need to harness the strategies you have learned in previous chapters. Notice the monsters that come out to play, and recognise their ugliness and noise for what it is: a trick. Notice the thoughts that come up and notice that they are just that: mere thoughts. Make room for the emotions that show up. Be present, in that very moment, as you 'do' becoming the mum you want to be.

Anxiety

A type of pain that you'll probably encounter as you move in the right direction is anxiety. A rush of anxiety is a sign that something is happening that matters to you. We don't tend to worry about things that don't matter. At times, the way to protect the thing that matters to you is to avoid the danger. For example, a childless friend unknowingly offers to give yourself and baby a lift in her car with you holding the baby, thinking that the lack of a capsule won't matter for a short trip. You experience a rush of panic, with horrible visions of baby being propelled through the windshield, and decide to protect the thing that matters to you—your baby—by taking your own car instead.

Avoidance is a natural response to many anxiety-provoking situations, but it isn't always helpful. At other times the way to protect the thing that matters to you isn't about avoiding the 'danger'. There is a certain level of danger—of risk—that is a part of life and cannot be fully avoided. In our example above, although the mum decided to take her own car instead of going with her friend, she was still exposed to the risk of a potential car crash (after all, she didn't decide to remain housebound). There are also 'dangers' that we spend time trying to avoid when they aren't actually dangers at all—because they don't really exist—such as our thoughts and feelings. For example, a new mum may feel highly anxious about taking her baby out for the first time. She may experience a rush of panic and horrible visions of herself covered in baby poo, of other people criticising how she feeds or of her baby screaming. It may be tempting to never step outside again in order to avoid the anxious feelings and horrible thoughts, but doing so won't help her to become the mum she wants to be.

Step by step

If a particular goal or a specific action that you want to take as a mum causes a real rush of anxiety, or causes your monsters to become quite ugly and noisy, it is possible to break the goal into smaller steps and take them one at a time. So, for example, the woman who feels a rush of anxiety about taking her baby out may decide to approach the outing in steps like this:

1 Take baby to visit my parents with my partner.
2 Take baby to visit my parents alone.
3 Take baby to visit the shops with my partner or my parents.
4 Take baby to visit the shops with a supportive friend.
5 Take baby to visit the shops alone for a quick trip.
6 Take baby to visit the shops alone and actually do some shopping.

By breaking down goals in this way they become more manageable, realistic and achievable. The idea is that you keep moving in the direction in which you want to go, but you just take smaller steps. It is okay for each step to be very small, but every time you take a step you must really take it. In other words, for every step, be fully present.

Think small

It is important that, in addition to the larger goals that you may set, you also think small. Larger goals are great, but what babies really need are the little acts of love, repeated consistently over and over, day by day. Remember, a truly small act is something that is easy for you to do and that doesn't require much effort or time.

Small mothering acts (once baby is born) might include:

- ✩ giving baby a kiss
- ✩ giving baby a cuddle
- ✩ feeding baby
- ✩ holding baby
- ✩ lying baby beside you
- ✩ having baby with you in a sling/possum pouch
- ✩ smiling at baby
- ✩ singing to baby
- ✩ talking to baby
- ✩ noticing what baby is doing
- ✩ playing with baby
- ✩ taking baby for a walk
- ✩ showing baby something she will find interesting
- ✩ giving baby an opportunity to learn, such as tummy time.

Notice that some of these acts may not always be small; for example, holding baby may be a small act when baby is quiet and a big act when baby is crying. Also, some acts may be small for some women and big for others; for example, some women may find singing to their baby easy and natural, while others may find it challenging even though they strongly value it. It is important then to think about small acts for you, given your mothering values.

What are some little ways in which you can live your mothering values once your baby is born?

....

....

....

....

....

Now that you have a list of small acts, think about how you can build these acts into your day. You might like to consider building some of these acts into your daily routines. For example, you could make sure that you talk to your baby every time you change his nappy, or you could sing to your baby when you dress him, or you might decide to cuddle your baby during his afternoon nap. Attaching these small acts to aspects of your daily routine as a new mum makes it easier to ensure that you start doing them. As you do them regularly you will find that these acts become more and more natural. You can also consider putting your list of acts somewhere visible, such as on the fridge, to remind yourself of them.

SMALL ACTS FOR HERE AND NOW

If you aren't yet a new mum, you may need to be creative in applying your values here and now. Some mothering acts, such as talking and singing to baby and noticing baby, can begin during pregnancy. Beginning to incorporate these acts into your daily life during pregnancy can create strong habits for when baby is born. If you have a richer understanding of your values as a mum, and the many and varied ways in which you can live out those values, then it is easier to be creative and to find ways of being the mum that you want to be in a variety of different circumstances. For example, if your baby is born pre-term and needs to spend time in the neonatal intensive care unit at hospital, you may find that many of the things that you were expecting to be able to do for your baby, such as cuddle her, feed her or bath her, you cannot do straight away. If you have a richer understanding of your values it is easier to find the ways that you can be the mum that you want to be for your baby; for example, by talking and singing to her.

Finding ways of living out your values as a mum may be even more challenging while you are waiting to conceive (especially if you are having difficulty) or if you experience a miscarriage or stillbirth. While waiting to conceive, consider ways that you can prepare for your future baby; for example, if you plan on singing your baby lots of lullabies then you may enjoy taking singing lessons while you wait to fall pregnant. You may also find other ways to live out your mothering values beyond your anticipated role as a mother; for example, in your relationships with children in your wider family or friendship circle.

If you have experienced a miscarriage or stillbirth, then consider how you can honour your lost baby or babies. There are many different ways to honour lost babies, and you should choose what feels right for you. Some options that women choose include ceremonies such as lighting a candle, planting a tree or garden, making baby a toy or piece of clothing, making a keepsake box, carrying a keepsake such as keepsake jewellery, cuddling a doll or teddy bear or framing photos. Remember that there is no one right way to grieve, so you should do what feels right for you. A woman will always be mum to the babies that she has lost. You should feel free to find ways for you to be the mum that you want to be to your lost babies, too.

What are some *small* acts I can do right now to be the mum that I want to be?

....

....

....

....

....

....

EXPECT TO SLIP

It is inevitable that when we try to make changes in our behaviour, we will slip and make mistakes. We are, after all, only human. So, expect to slip. Becoming the mum that you want to be is not about not slipping; it is about what you do after you slip. Just after you've slipped your monsters will probably be very ugly and very noisy. They will try to convince you to give up. Expect this to happen. Be prepared to notice that it is simply your monsters talking. Notice that your thoughts at this time are just thoughts. Are you able to make room for this mistake and keep moving towards being the mum that you want to be?

As we saw earlier, you become the mum that you want to be through the accumulation of many small acts. The marvellous thing about this is that there is actually a lot of room for mistakes. So a woman becomes a loving mum by building up a million tiny acts of love. She'll become that loving mum regardless of how affectionate she was on a particular Tuesday when her baby was three weeks old. To be a loving mum you don't need to be loving absolutely all of the time in every possible way; you just need to be loving enough. There is space for bad moments and mistakes, space for you to be human.

DO WHAT WORKS IN BECOMING THE MUM YOU WANT TO BE

Your values are your guiding stars. They set your course and help you to determine your goals as a mum and the actions that you'll take as a mum moment by moment and day by day. Ensure that your mothering values aren't sidelined by the *It shouldn't be like this* monster. This monster will try to convince you that you'll enjoy motherhood more if you could only fix all of the 'problems' with yourself and with your baby. If you get cornered by this monster you'll notice yourself setting mothering goals that aren't based on your values or becoming the mum that you want to be but, rather, are based on trying to 'fix' your baby. You'll also probably find that much of what you are trying to do isn't working.

How you are as a mum should also be determined by doing what works for you, considering how your baby actually is, in the context of your values. Thinking about what is effective is a continuous process. Get into the habit of regularly evaluating whether the actions that you are taking as a mum are working, in accordance with your values. If your actions aren't working, experiment until you find what does work for you and your baby, in line with your values. This makes you flexible in your mothering.

For example, a mum might strongly value reading to her baby and may decide to read a book to her baby every evening as part of the bedtime ritual. She might find, however, that her baby is unsettled in the evening and that this doesn't work. It therefore doesn't work in terms of her values either, as she isn't enjoying reading to her baby and she doesn't feel that she is effectively encouraging a love of books or language development, as her baby is just too unsettled to take it in. She may then decide to read her baby a book in the mornings instead.

This idea of doing what works may seem very simple, but it can be easy to get stuck in a cycle of repeating actions that don't work because we are attached to our plans and our goals. In other words, we may keep pushing for our baby and our mothering experience to fit what we expected it to be like, instead of allowing our baby and our experience to be what it is.

ACTUALLY DOING IT

Pick some *small* acts that you can put into practice right now to be the mum that you want to be, and do them today. Notice the effects of this.

Did you enjoy taking these steps? Did your monsters become noisy? If you noticed your monsters, how can you use the strategies in this book to ensure that you keep moving in the right direction?

....

....

....

....

....

....

....

ONE WOMAN'S STORY

Reading Leila's story may help you to live out your own values as a mum.

Leila gave birth to her twins Harry and Sophie when she was 30 weeks pregnant. Leila and her partner Justin had been advised that there was an increased chance of premature labour with twins, but it was still a shock when it actually happened to them. They found that having both multiples and babies born prematurely made it more challenging to adapt to parenthood.

Leila found it heart wrenching that she was discharged from hospital while her twins, due to their prematurity, had to stay. Her first weeks of motherhood simply weren't what she had thought they would be, and it was challenging to find ways to mother within a hospital environment. However, she connected with her values as a mum and was creative in finding ways to live these values, as best she could, while her babies were in hospital. In particular, Leila found that singing and talking to her babies was very important. She could sing and talk to her babies even in the early days when it wasn't possible to hold them. Leila would listen to children's music and lullabies when she was at home so that she could learn more songs to sing to Harry and Sophie. This made her feel like she was still doing something for her babies, even while she was between hospital visits. Leila would bring children's books into the hospital when she visited, and read them to the twins. Sometimes she would just talk about the details of her day. It felt good to be able to do something that was important to her as a mum.

When Leila and Justin first brought the babies home it was thrilling but also nerve racking. Harry and Sophie had been so vulnerable when they were first born that Leila was understandably anxious about them. In addition, she had become used to mothering with a nurse always a call away, so it was frightening to suddenly find herself with full responsibility for the twins. Justin was supportive but had long since returned to work.

At first, Leila felt overwhelmed. She then decided that she would identify the tasks that she found most scary and to take them step by step. One task that she found particularly unnerving was bathing Harry and Sophie, so Leila decided that she would begin by bathing the babies in the evenings when Justin could help out. Once Leila felt comfortable bathing the twins with assistance from Justin, she began to bath Harry and Sophie on her own, but at a time when Justin was still in the house. That way, if she needed back-up she could easily call for him. Finally, she began to bath baby Harry and baby Sophie during the day when Justin was at work.

Breaking down any frightening tasks into small steps made them less daunting. Within a couple of months Leila felt comfortable and confident with her babies.

MY UNIQUE ADVENTURE
These comments may help you to understand how the information in this chapter might relate to your unique experience.

Reversing the downward spiral
May be relevant to women with a history of depression, at risk of postnatal depression or experiencing postnatal depression.
Building a rewarding life is a vital part of treating and preventing depression. An important part of this is finding what is rewarding in your new life as a mum. Experiment with the small actions you can take to be the mum that you want to be. Do some of these actions give you a feeling of satisfaction or bring you joy? If so, repeat!

Grief and loss
May be relevant to any woman experiencing a loss, whether it be an obvious loss such as miscarriage or stillbirth, or the loss of pre-motherhood life, difficulty conceiving, an unwanted birth experience or motherhood being different from expectations.
If you have experienced a miscarriage or stillbirth, you may find it helpful to find ways in which you can honour your lost

baby. Are there actions you'd like to take to express your mothering values towards your baby? You may like to consider ideas like writing him a letter or poem, planting a tree, lighting a candle, keeping photos, or buying or making a keepsake such as a teddy bear or pendant. Be creative and find something that has meaning for you. There is no 'right' way to grieve. You will always be Mum to your babies, and you should feel free to continue to mother your babies in ways that feel right for you. It is also important to consider how you can best honour your baby in how you continue to live your life day by day. All babies deserve a mum who takes care of herself.

How do I survive this?

May be relevant to women experiencing emotional challenges, tough physical symptoms such as morning sickness, or birth.

The challenging times are when it is most important to think small. Remember that a truly small action is one that is easy to do, even on the bad days. What are the tiny things that you can do towards becoming the mum you want to be? During the challenging times this may be as simple as continuing to live through the challenge, moment by moment.

Living with worry and anxiety

May be relevant to women with a history of anxiety, women struggling with anxiety or worries, or women with a specific worry about motherhood.

When you begin taking steps towards being the mum you want to be, anxiety is likely to appear. You may need to be willing to experience anxiety to achieve your goals and become the mother that you want to be. You can approach goals that are anxiety provoking by breaking them into small steps and taking them one at a time. Remember that though you can make each step as small as you like, when you take the step you need to be willing to truly take it, and also to experience the anxiety that this may trigger.

PUTTING IT INTO PRACTICE

✩ If there are goals that you'd like to set for yourself, or actions that you'd like to take, that make you feel particularly anxious or overwhelmed, break these down into smaller steps. Would it be less overwhelming to have a support person with you at first? Or is there a smaller version of the action that you could take to begin with? Remember that you can make each step as small as you like, but when you take a step, take it fully.

✩ Write a list of small acts that you can take now, at your current stage of the motherhood journey. You may need to be creative. Consider if there is anything that you could do now to prepare for your baby. If you are currently pregnant, consider reconnecting with your values and making your baby the focus of living through the physical challenges of pregnancy.

✩ When you are acting based on your values you'll often notice a feeling of satisfaction or enjoyment. This doesn't mean that it is always easy, but only that acting on one's values feels right. Develop a habit of looking for that feeling and noticing what you are doing at the time. What value is that action based on? Can you repeat it?

✩ Develop a habit of considering whether what you are doing with your baby is working. That is, is what you are doing with your baby taking you closer to being the mum that you want to be?

16

In a
nutshell

Every word of this book, every exercise, every change you've made so far is all about this: becoming the mum that you want to be. It is about how you become a mother, little by little, day by day, moment by moment. This is your journey. Why are you doing any of this? The answer is simple. You are doing it for your baby. In this chapter we summarise how you can use the strategies of this book moment by moment as you continue with your journey and become the mum that you want to be.

THIS IS YOUR ADVENTURE

Becoming Mum has the potential to be one of the most rewarding, satisfying and exciting journeys of a woman's life. It is also frightening, sad, painful and overwhelming. Your adventure is uniquely your own. I don't know how your journey has unfolded so far or how it will continue to unfold. There are many aspects of your adventure that you yourself cannot control, from how long it will take you to conceive, to how your pregnancy unfolds, to the birth experience that you have, to who exactly your baby is. Scary, huh? But it is also part of what makes the voyage worth taking.

There are two ways to take this adventure. You can take it determined to not feel pain, making your very actions as a mum about avoiding the fears and sadness and unknowingly missing out on the joy too. Or you can take it bravely, with a heart wide open to the experience and to your baby. Yes, at times you will feel frightened, sad or disappointed; at times you will think scary thoughts, and at times you will make mistakes. It is about accepting all of that and becoming the mum that you want to be, remembering that becoming the mum that you want to be is a million little somethings that you *do* and that you can start doing right now.

THE JOURNEY IN A MOMENT

In one moment you can remember to become the mum that *you* want to be by remembering these four steps:

1 Anchoring:
  Anchor yourself in the here and now.
  Anchor yourself in your values as a mum.

2 Awareness:
  Expand your awareness in the here and now.
  Notice your thoughts as thoughts.
  Notice your feelings as feelings.
  Notice your baby as she is in the here and now.

3 Acceptance:
  Make room for your own thoughts and feelings.
  Become an accepting space for baby as she is in the here and now.
  Find kindness for yourself.
  Find kindness for baby.

4 Action:
  Take action based on your values (remember that it can be *small*).
  Follow up by asking whether your actions are *working* (in accordance with your values).

Depending on what is unfolding for you in that moment, you may emphasise different aspects of the four steps; for example, in one moment the main task may be finding kindness for yourself, whereas in another it may be getting in contact with your values.

You also may use different strategies from this book in order to do this. The strategies covered in this book may fit into the four steps like this:

1 **Anchoring:**
Anchor yourself in the here and now.
Anchor yourself in your values as a mum.
This might involve:
✩ mindfulness of breathing
✩ mindfulness of your current activity
✩ mindfulness of baby
✩ reminding yourself of your values.

2 **Awareness:**
Expand your awareness in the here and now.
Notice your thoughts as thoughts.
Notice your feelings as feelings.
Notice your baby as she is in the here and now.
This might involve:
✩ mindfulness of breathing
✩ mindfulness of your current activity
✩ mindfulness of baby
✩ mindfulness of emotions
✩ mindfulness of thoughts.

3 **Acceptance:**
Make room for your own thoughts and feelings.
Become an accepting space for baby as she is in the here and now.
Find kindness for yourself.
Find kindness for baby.
This might involve:

☆ mindfulness of emotions
☆ mindfulness of thoughts
☆ becoming an accepting space
☆ self-kindness
☆ kindness for baby.

4 **Action:**

Take action based on your values (remember that it can be *small*). Follow up by asking whether your actions are *working* (in accordance with your values).

This might involve:

☆ acting on your values as a mum
☆ acting on one of your other values
☆ connecting with your partner
☆ an act of self-kindness
☆ getting support.

TAKE THIS LIGHTLY TOO!

If you've truly taken in the message of this book you'll know that you shouldn't live your life by the advice in this book. In other words, don't turn the concepts of this book, such as being mindful, into just another monster. Remember that the thought 'I'm not practising mindfulness enough' is also just a thought, and sadness at not accepting your emotions is just another emotion to make room for. So don't start steering your ship by the words in this book; steer it by what you've always had in your heart. Steer your ship by your guiding stars—your values—and alter your course as necessary along the way so that you are doing what works for you and for your baby.

As you continue on your voyage I guarantee that you'll slip. When you do so, try as best you can to make room for your mistake. And when you slip at that too, be kind to yourself.

AND FINALLY ...

Becoming Mum has the potential to be deeply rewarding, satisfying and joyful. This is *your* journey. Enjoy it.

A POEM FOR BABY

Fill my heart with your sorrows
and I shall hold them
Fill my life with your needs
and I shall meet them
Fill my spirit with your joy
and I shall embrace it
with a reckless abandon
With a heart wide open
to all your possibilities
With room for your sorrows
and room for your joy
Room enough for all of it
With an unrelenting, bottomless passion
I love you

A SECOND POEM FOR BABY

And I promise you this
I will make mistakes
Glorious, massive mistakes
And I will make room for them
so that I can make room
for your mistakes
Your glorious, massive mistakes
There's room enough in my heart
for all of both of us
There's no need for either of us
to cut ourselves to bits
And I promise you this
I will make your joyful flourishing
your glorious, joyful flourishing
my first priority
There's room enough
for that, too

What is the research behind this book?

This book is based on the latest research in developmental and clinical psychology.

The therapeutic approach in this book is based on the newest developments in Cognitive Behavioural Therapy (CBT), including Acceptance and Commitment Therapy (ACT, said as one word: 'ACT') (Hayes, Strosahl, & Wilson, 2003) and mindfulness-based Cognitive Behavioural Therapy. Concepts and exercises adapted from ACT (Hayes, 2004; Hayes, Luoma, Bond, Masuda, & Lillis, 2006; Hayes et al., 2003) are covered in depth in Chapters 1-3, 6-8 and 14-15, including the importance of basing your actions on your unique mothering values, the concept that joy and emotional pain are attached, the futility of struggling with emotional pain, and the concepts of living with your monsters as they are, getting distance from your thoughts, accepting your emotions and committing yourself to action.

Further, the overall approach of this book, from start to finish, is grounded within the ACT therapeutic approach. ACT has a growing evidence base, with systematic literature reviews of ACT concluding that it is effective (Hayes, et al., 2006; Ost, 2008; Ruiz, 2010, 2012). The mindfulness exercises in Chapters 4-6 and Chapter 8—including mindfulness of breathing, mindfulness of eating, mindfulness of walking, mindfulness in everyday life, mindfulness of baby, mindfulness of thoughts and mindfulness of pain—were adapted for mothers from mindfulness exercises used within mindfulness-based CBT, including Mindfulness Based Stress Reduction (MBSR) (Kabat-Zinn, 1990) and Mindfulness Based Cognitive Therapy (MBCT) (Segal, Teasdale, & Williams, 2004; Segal, Williams, & Teasdale, 2002).

In addition, adaption was made with an understanding of mindfulness as it has been practised for thousands of years within Buddhist meditative traditions (Kang & Whittingham, 2010). There is a growing evidence base for the therapeutic benefits of mindfulness for a range of clinical conditions, including depression and anxiety, as well as for improving one's ability to cope with the general stresses of everyday life and improving psychological functioning (Grossman, Niemann, Schmidt, & Walach, 2004; Baer, 2003; Baer et al., 2008; Coelho, Canter, & Ernst, 2007). Chapter 10, on taking care of yourself, in addition to drawing upon ACT, also draws upon Compassionate Mind Training in developing relevant exercises to cultivate self-kindness and defuse self-criticism (Gilbert & Procter, 2006). In Chapter 11 the benefits of building a rewarding life are discussed. This draws directly from Behavioural Activation (or Pleasant Events Scheduling), an evidence-based therapy for depression in its own right that normally forms a part of any CBT for depression (Jacobson, Martell, & Dimidjian, 2001).

This book is also grounded in developmental psychology; in particular, understanding that healthy infant development always occurs within the context of attachment bonds with caregivers (Bowlby, 1988). Infant development is fundamentally an interpersonal process (Ainsworth, Blehar, Waters & Wall, 1978; Bowlby, 1988; Siegel, 2012; Sroufe, 2005). This view of infancy, coupled with an ACT therapeutic approach, provided the basis for this book. In particular, Chapter 9, on loving baby, draws upon Attachment Theory, including the advice that a strong attachment bond with baby is best built through sensitive and responsive mothering (Ainsworth, Blehar, Waters & Wall, 1978; Sroufe, 2005).

In Chapter 14 there is a section on understanding your newborn baby. This section draws upon current research on babies in claiming the following:

Human newborns are developmentally like foetuses. In fact, the evidence suggests that human evolution has necessitated humans giving birth to 'premature' infants as the only way for humans to both have large brains and walk upright (Buck, 2011). This suggests that human newborns should not be expected to show independence and should, in fact, be parented so that they receive responsiveness to their needs and physical comfort that is similar to that which they would receive if they were still living in the uterus. Putting infant behaviour into this neurodevelopmental context, it is likely that a newborn infant's intense emotional reactions, high needs for comfort and night-time waking are all developmentally normal.

Maternal responsiveness and sensitivity is important for later psychological health. Maternal responsiveness and sensitivity involves a mother recognising the emotions and needs of her infant and, as best she can, sensitively responding to those needs. Maternal responsiveness and sensitivity during infancy is associated with a secure attachment bond between the infant and the mother at 12 and 18 months of age (Sroufe, 2005). Toddlers with secure attachment use their caregivers as a secure base for exploration, confidently exploring their environment and learning while maintaining proximity to their caregiver. Toddlers with secure attachment also use their caregivers as a safe haven for comfort, approaching them when distressed and settling well with responsive parenting. Secure attachment predicts later social competence, emotional regulation abilities and independence.

It is normal for infants to seek comfort from their attachment figures when they are distressed or in need of emotional or behavioural regulation. This seeking of comfort for emotional regulation is a normal element of a healthy and secure attachment bond. As infants' brains are still maturing, they rely upon input from caregivers to regulate their emotions and behaviour (Siegel, 2012). High dependency on caregivers in infancy doesn't predict later dependency in childhood, if the dependency needs are met (Sroufe, 2005). In fact, if the dependency needs are met, it predicts greater independence.

Night wakings are common (and thus, may well be part of normal variation in infants). As many as one third of infants continue to wake during the night at their first birthday, and the majority of these infants start sleeping through the night before their second birthday (Weinraub et al., 2012).

References

Ainsworth, M.D.S., Blehar, M.C., Waters, E., & Wall, S. (1978). *Patterns of attachment. A psychological study of the strange situation.* New Jersey: Lawrence Erlbaum Associates.

Baer, R. A. (2003). Mindfulness training as a clinical intervention: A conceptual and empirical review. *Clinical Psychology: Science and Practice*, 10 (2), 125–143.

Baer, R. A., Smith, G. T., Lykins, E., Button, D., Krietemeyer, J., & Sauer, S., et al. (2008). Construct validity of the Five Facet Mindfulness Questionnaire in meditating and non-meditating samples. Assessment, 15, 329–342.

Bowlby, J. (1988). *A secure base: Parent–child attachment and healthy human development.* New York: Basic Books.

Buck, S. (2011). The evolutionary history of the modern birth mechanism: looking at skeletal and cultural adaptations. *Totem: the University of Western Ontario Journal of Anthropology*, 19 (1), 81–91.

Carmody, J., & Baer, R. A. (2008). Relationships between mindfulness practice and levels of mindfulness, medical and psychological symptoms and well-being in a mindfulness-based stress reduction program. *Journal of Behavioural Medicine*, 31, 23–33.

Coelho, H. F., Canter, R. H., & Ernst, E. (2007). Mindfulness-based cognitive therapy: Evaluating current evidence and informing future research. *Journal of Consulting and Clinical Psychology*, 75 (6), 1000–1005.

Gilbert, P., & Procter, S. (2006). Compassionate mind training for people with high shame and self-criticism: Overview and pilot study of a group therapy approach. *Clinical Psychology and Psychotherapy*, 13, 353–379.

Grossman, P., Niemann, L., Schmidt, S., & Walach, H. (2004). Mindfulness-based stress reduction and health benefits: A meta-analysis. *Journal of Psychosomatic Research*, 57, 35–43.

Hayes, S. C. (2004). Acceptance and Commitment Therapy and the new behavior therapies. In S. C. Hayes, V. M. Follette & M. M. Linehan (Eds.), *Mindfulness and acceptance expanding the cognitive-behavioral tradition*. New York: The Guilford Press.

Hayes, S. C., Luoma, J. B., Bond, F. W., Masuda, A., & Lillis, J. (2006). Acceptance and Commitment Therapy: Model, processes and outcomes. *Behaviour Research and Therapy*, 44, 1–25.

Hayes, S. C., Strosahl, K. D., & Wilson, K. G. (2003). *Acceptance and Commitment Therapy: An experiential approach to behavior change*. New York: The Guilford Press.

Jacobson, N. S., Martell, C. R., & Dimidjian, S. (2001). Behavioural Activation for depression: Returning to contextual roots. *Clinical Psychology: Science and Practice*, 8 (3), 255–270.

Kabat-Zinn, J. (1990). *Full catastrophe living: How to cope with stress, pain and illness using mindfulness meditation*. New York: Dell Publishing.

Kang, C., & Whittingham, K. (2010). Mindfulness: A dialogue between Buddhism and clinical psychology. *Mindfulness*, 1 (3), 161–173.

Ost, L. (2008). Efficacy of the third wave of behavioral therapies: A systematic review and meta-analysis. *Behaviour Research and Therapy*, 46, 296–321.

Ruiz, F. J. (2010). A review of Acceptance and Commitment therapy (ACT) empirical evidence: correlational, experimental psychopathology, component and outcome studies. *International Journal of Psychology and Psychological Therapy*, 10 (1), 125–162.

Ruiz, F. J. (2012). Acceptance and Commitment Therapy versus Traditional Cognitive Behavioral Therapy: A systematic review and meta-analysis of current empirical evidence. *International Journal of Psychology and Psychological Therapy*, 12 (3), 333–358.

Segal, Z. V., Teasdale, J. D., & Williams, M. G. (2004). Mindfulness-Based Cognitive Therapy. In S. C. Hayes, V. M. Follette & M. M. Linehan (Eds.), *Mindfulness and acceptance expanding the cognitive-behavioral tradition*. New York: The Guilford Press.

Segal, Z. V., Williams, J. M. G., & Teasdale, J. D. (2002). *Mindfulness-Based Cognitive Therapy for depression a new approach to preventing relapse*. New York: The Guilford Press.

Siegel, D. J. (2012). *The developing mind: How relationships and the brain interact to shape who we are* (2nd edn). New York: The Guilford Press.

Sroufe, A. L. (2005). Attachment and development: A prospective, longitudinal study from birth to adulthood. *Attachment and Human Development*, 7 (4), 349–367.

Weinraub, M., Bender, R. H., Friedman, S. L., Susman, E. J., Knoke, B., Bradley, R., et al. (2012). Patterns of developmental change in infants' nighttime sleep awakenings from 6 through 36 months of age. *Developmental Psychology*. 48 (6), 1511–1528.

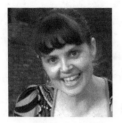

About the author

Dr Koa Whittingham is a psychologist with specialisations in both clinical and developmental psychology. She is a research fellow at the Queensland Cerebral Palsy and Rehabilitation Research Centre at The University of Queensland, where she conducts research on parenting, neurodevelopmental disabilities, Acceptance and Commitment Therapy and mindfulness. In July 2011, Koa fulfilled a lifelong dream by giving birth to her first child and becoming a mum. Koa wrote *Becoming Mum* while she was on maternity leave, with much of the content quite literally written while her beloved baby slept on her chest.

Koa regularly writes about parenting isues on her blog, Parenting from the Heart.

koawhittingham.com

Printed in Australia
AUOC02n1312251113
258794AU00012B/12/P